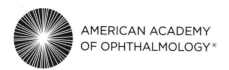

AMERICAN ACADEMY
OF OPHTHALMOLOGY®

MW00427518

Glaucoma

Last major revision 2016–2017

2019–2020
BCSC

Basic and Clinical
Science Course™

Protecting Sight. Empowering Lives.®

EB○ Published after collaborative
review with the European Board
of Ophthalmology subcommittee

The American Academy of Ophthalmology is accredited by the Accreditation Council for Continuing Medical Education (ACCME) to provide continuing medical education for physicians.

The American Academy of Ophthalmology designates this enduring material for a maximum of 10 *AMA PRA Category 1 Credits*™. Physicians should claim only the credit commensurate with the extent of their participation in the activity.

Originally released June 2016; reviewed for currency September 2018; CME expiration date: June 1, 2020. *AMA PRA Category 1 Credits*™ may be claimed only once between June 1, 2016, and the expiration date.

BCSC® volumes are designed to increase the physician's ophthalmic knowledge through study and review. Users of this activity are encouraged to read the text and then answer the study questions provided at the back of the book.

To claim *AMA PRA Category 1 Credits*™ upon completion of this activity, learners must demonstrate appropriate knowledge and participation in the activity by taking the posttest for Section 10 and achieving a score of 80% or higher. For further details, please see the instructions for requesting CME credit at the back of the book.

The Academy provides this material for educational purposes only. It is not intended to represent the only or best method or procedure in every case, nor to replace a physician's own judgment or give specific advice for case management. Including all indications, contraindications, side effects, and alternative agents for each drug or treatment is beyond the scope of this material. All information and recommendations should be verified, prior to use, with current information included in the manufacturers' package inserts or other independent sources, and considered in light of the patient's condition and history. Reference to certain drugs, instruments, and other products in this course is made for illustrative purposes only and is not intended to constitute an endorsement of such. Some material may include information on applications that are not considered community standard, that reflect indications not included in approved FDA labeling, or that are approved for use only in restricted research settings. **The FDA has stated that it is the responsibility of the physician to determine the FDA status of each drug or device he or she wishes to use, and to use them with appropriate, informed patient consent in compliance with applicable law.** The Academy specifically disclaims any and all liability for injury or other damages of any kind, from negligence or otherwise, for any and all claims that may arise from the use of any recommendations or other information contained herein.

All trademarks, trade names, logos, brand names, and service marks of the American Academy of Ophthalmology (AAO), whether registered or unregistered, are the property of AAO and are protected by US and international trademark laws. These trademarks include AAO; AAOE; AMERICAN ACADEMY OF OPHTHALMOLOGY; BASIC AND CLINICAL SCIENCE COURSE; BCSC; EYENET; EYEWIKI; FOCAL POINTS; FOCUS DESIGN (logo shown on cover); IRIS; ISRS; OKAP; ONE NETWORK; OPHTHALMOLOGY; OPHTHALMOLOGY GLAUCOMA; OPHTHALMOLOGY RETINA; PREFERRED PRACTICE PATTERN; PROTECTING SIGHT. EMPOWERING LIVES; and THE OPHTHALMIC NEWS & EDUCATION NETWORK.

Cover image: From BCSC Section 9, *Uveitis and Ocular Inflammation.* Large mutton-fat keratic precipitates in a patient with sarcoidosis. *(Courtesy of Debra Goldstein, MD.)*

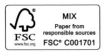

Printed in China.

Basic and Clinical Science Course

Louis B. Cantor, MD, Indianapolis, Indiana, *Senior Secretary for Clinical Education*

Christopher J. Rapuano, MD, Philadelphia, Pennsylvania, *Secretary for Lifelong Learning and Assessment*

Colin A. McCannel, MD, Los Angeles, California, *BCSC Course Chair*

Section 10

Faculty for the Major Revision

Christopher A. Girkin, MD, *Chair,* Birmingham, Alabama

Anjali M. Bhorade, MD, St Louis, Missouri

Jonathan G. Crowston, MBBS, PhD, East Melbourne, Victoria, Australia

JoAnn A. Giaconi, MD, Los Angeles, California

Felipe A. Medeiros, MD, PhD, San Diego, California

Arthur J. Sit, MD, Rochester, Minnesota

Angelo P. Tanna, MD, Chicago, Illinois

The Academy wishes to acknowledge the *American Glaucoma Society* for recommending faculty members to the BCSC Section 10 committee.

The Academy also wishes to acknowledge the following committees for review of this edition:

Committee on Aging: Thomas A. Graul, MD, Lincoln, Nebraska

Vision Rehabilitation Committee: Paul I. Homer, MD, Boca Raton, Florida

Practicing Ophthalmologists Advisory Committee for Education: James A. Savage, MD, *Primary Reviewer,* Memphis, Tennessee; Edward K. Isbey III, MD, *Chair,* Asheville, North Carolina; Alice Bashinsky, MD, Asheville, North Carolina; David Browning, MD, PhD, Charlotte, North Carolina; Bradley Fouraker, MD, Tampa, Florida; Dasa Gangadhar, MD, Wichita, Kansas; Steven J. Grosser, MD, Golden Valley, Minnesota; Stephen R. Klapper, MD, Carmel, Indiana

European Board of Ophthalmology: Carlo Traverso, MD, *Chair,* Genoa, Italy; Gordana Sunaric Mégevand, MD, FMH, FEBO, *Liaison,* Geneva, Switzerland; Augusto Azuara-Blanco, PhD, FRCS(Ed), FRCOphth, Belfast, Northern Ireland; Anders Heijl, MD, PhD, Malmö, Sweden; Gabor Hollo, MD, PhD, DSc, Budapest, Hungary; Anja Tuulonen, MD, PhD, Tampere, Finland

Financial Disclosures

The other authors and reviewers state that within the 12 months prior to their contributions to this CME activity and for the duration of development, they have had no financial interest in or other relationship with any entity discussed in this course that produces, markets, resells, or distributes ophthalmic health care goods or services consumed by or used in patients, or with any competing commercial product or service.

Recent Past Faculty

Keith Barton, MD
George A. Cioffi, MD
F. Jane Durcan, MD
Neeru Gupta, MD, PhD
Jody R. Piltz-Seymour, MD
Thomas W. Samuelson, MD

In addition, the Academy gratefully acknowledges the contributions of numerous past faculty and advisory committee members who have played an important role in the development of previous editions of the Basic and Clinical Science Course.

American Academy of Ophthalmology Staff

Dale E. Fajardo, EdD, MBA, *Vice President, Education*
Beth Wilson, *Director, Continuing Professional Development*
Ann McGuire, *Acquisitions and Development Manager*
Stephanie Tanaka, *Publications Manager*
D. Jean Ray, *Production Manager*
Beth Collins, *Medical Editor*
Naomi Ruiz, *Publications Specialist*

American Academy of Ophthalmology
655 Beach Street
Box 7424
San Francisco, CA 94120-7424

Contents

General Introduction

The Basic and Clinical Science Course (BCSC) is designed to meet the needs of residents and practitioners for a comprehensive yet concise curriculum of the field of ophthalmology. The BCSC has developed from its original brief outline format, which relied heavily on outside readings, to a more convenient and educationally useful self-contained text. The Academy updates and revises the course annually, with the goals of integrating the basic science and clinical practice of ophthalmology and of keeping ophthalmologists current with new developments in the various subspecialties.

The BCSC incorporates the effort and expertise of more than 90 ophthalmologists, organized into 13 Section faculties, working with Academy editorial staff. In addition, the course continues to benefit from many lasting contributions made by the faculties of previous editions. Members of the Academy Practicing Ophthalmologists Advisory Committee for Education, Committee on Aging, and Vision Rehabilitation Committee review every volume before major revisions. Members of the European Board of Ophthalmology, organized into Section faculties, also review each volume before major revisions, focusing primarily on differences between American and European ophthalmology practice.

Organization of the Course

The Basic and Clinical Science Course comprises 13 volumes, incorporating fundamental ophthalmic knowledge, subspecialty areas, and special topics:

1 Update on General Medicine
2 Fundamentals and Principles of Ophthalmology
3 Clinical Optics
4 Ophthalmic Pathology and Intraocular Tumors
5 Neuro-Ophthalmology
6 Pediatric Ophthalmology and Strabismus
7 Oculofacial Plastic and Orbital Surgery
8 External Disease and Cornea
9 Uveitis and Ocular Inflammation
10 Glaucoma
11 Lens and Cataract
12 Retina and Vitreous
13 Refractive Surgery

In addition, a comprehensive Master Index allows the reader to easily locate subjects throughout the entire series.

References

Readers who wish to explore specific topics in greater detail may consult the references cited within each chapter and listed in the Basic Texts section at the back of the book.

These references are intended to be selective rather than exhaustive, chosen by the BCSC faculty as being important, current, and readily available to residents and practitioners.

Multimedia

This edition of Section 10, *Glaucoma,* includes videos related to topics covered in the book. The videos were selected by members of the BCSC faculty and are available to readers of the print and electronic versions of Section 10 (www.aao.org/bcscvideo_section10). Mobile-device users can scan the QR code below (a QR-code reader must already be installed on the device) to access the video content.

Self-Assessment and CME Credit

Each volume of the BCSC is designed as an independent study activity for ophthalmology residents and practitioners. The learning objectives for this volume are given on page 1. The text, illustrations, and references provide the information necessary to achieve the objectives; the study questions allow readers to test their understanding of the material and their mastery of the objectives. Physicians who wish to claim CME credit for this educational activity may do so by following the instructions given at the end of the book.

This Section of the BCSC has been approved by the American Board of Ophthalmology as a Maintenance of Certification Part II self-assessment CME activity.

Conclusion

The Basic and Clinical Science Course has expanded greatly over the years, with the addition of much new text, numerous illustrations, and video content. Recent editions have sought to place greater emphasis on clinical applicability while maintaining a solid foundation in basic science. As with any educational program, it reflects the experience of its authors. As its faculties change and medicine progresses, new viewpoints emerge on controversial subjects and techniques. Not all alternate approaches can be included in this series; as with any educational endeavor, the learner should seek additional sources, including Academy Preferred Practice Pattern Guidelines.

The BCSC faculty and staff continually strive to improve the educational usefulness of the course; you, the reader, can contribute to this ongoing process. If you have any suggestions or questions about the series, please do not hesitate to contact the faculty or the editors.

The authors, editors, and reviewers hope that your study of the BCSC will be of lasting value and that each Section will serve as a practical resource for quality patient care.

Objectives

Upon completion of BCSC Section 10, *Glaucoma,* the reader should be able to

- state the epidemiologic features of glaucoma, including the social and economic impacts of the disease

- list recent advances in the understanding of hereditary and genetic factors in glaucoma

- describe the physiology of aqueous humor dynamics and the control of intraocular pressure (IOP)

- describe the clinical evaluation of the glaucoma patient, including history and general examination, gonioscopy, optic nerve examination, and visual field

- list the clinical features of the patient considered a glaucoma suspect

- describe the clinical features, evaluation, and treatment of primary open-angle glaucoma and normal-tension glaucoma

- list the various clinical features of and therapeutic approaches for the secondary open-angle glaucomas

- state the underlying causes of the increased IOP in various forms of secondary open-angle glaucoma and the impact that these underlying causes have on management

- describe the mechanisms and pathophysiology of primary angle-closure glaucoma

- describe the pathophysiology of secondary angle-closure glaucoma, both with and without pupillary block

- describe the pathophysiology of and therapy for primary congenital and juvenile-onset glaucomas

- describe the various classes of medical therapy for glaucoma, including efficacy, mechanism of action, and safety

- state the indications for, techniques used in, and complications of various laser and incisional surgical procedures for glaucoma

CHAPTER 1

Introduction to Glaucoma: Terminology, Epidemiology, and Heredity

Definitions

Glaucoma represents a group of diseases defined by a characteristic optic neuropathy that is consistent with remodeling of the connective tissue elements of the optic nerve head (also called the optic disc) and with loss of neural tissue associated with the eventual development of distinctive patterns of visual dysfunction. Although the *intraocular pressure (IOP)* level is one of the primary risk factors for development of glaucoma, it does not have a role in the definition of the disease; further, IOP of any level can have an impact on the risk of glaucoma.

Susceptibility to glaucoma is determined not only by the IOP, but also by the resilience of the optic nerve to the multiple pathogenic mechanisms involved in the neuropathy. Thus, in some individuals, progressive injury may occur at low IOP levels whereas in others with higher pressures, injury never occurs. When considering whether glaucomatous damage is truly occurring in a patient with "normal" IOP, the ophthalmologist should take into account measurement artifacts and circadian variations in IOP. In most cases of glaucoma, it is presumed that the IOP is too high for proper functioning of the optic nerve axons and that lowering the pressure will stabilize the damage. However, the optic nerve may continue to be damaged despite decreasing the IOP.

The term *preperimetric glaucoma* is sometimes used to denote glaucomatous changes in the optic nerve head in the absence of development of clinically detectable visual field damage.

Open-Angle, Angle-Closure, Primary, and Secondary Glaucomas

Traditionally, glaucoma has been classified as open-angle or angle-closure glaucoma and as primary or secondary (Table 1-1). Distinguishing open-angle glaucoma from angle-closure is essential from a therapeutic standpoint (Fig 1-1), and each type of glaucoma is discussed in detail in Chapters 4 and 5; normal aqueous humor flow in the eye is illustrated in Figure 1-2. The concept of primary and secondary glaucoma, while useful, reflects our lack of understanding of the pathophysiologic mechanisms underlying the glaucomatous process. Open-angle glaucoma is traditionally classified as primary when

Table 1-1 **Classification of the Glaucomas**

Type	Characteristics
Open-angle glaucoma and related diagnoses	
Primary open-angle glaucoma (POAG)	Not associated with known ocular or systemic disorders that cause increased resistance to aqueous outflow or damage to optic nerve; usually associated with elevated IOP
Normal-tension glaucoma (NTG)	Considered to be within the continuum of POAG; term often used when IOP is within the statistically normal range
Juvenile open-angle glaucoma (JOAG)	Term often used when open-angle glaucoma is diagnosed at a young age (typically 4–35 years of age)
Ocular hypertension (OHT)	Elevated IOP in the absence of optic nerve, retinal nerve fiber layer, or visual field abnormalities
Glaucoma suspect	Optic nerve head appearance or visual field suggestive of glaucoma regardless of IOP
Secondary open-angle glaucoma	Increased resistance to trabecular meshwork outflow associated with other conditions (eg, pigmentary, phacolytic, steroid-induced, pseudoexfoliation, angle-recession, and uveitic glaucomas)
	Elevated episcleral venous pressure (eg, carotid-cavernous sinus fistula, Sturge-Weber, idiopathic)
Angle-closure glaucoma (see Fig 1-1)	
Primary angle-closure suspect (PACS)	Narrow angle with no signs of trabecular meshwork or optic nerve damage
Primary angle closure (PAC)	Narrow angle with elevated IOP or PAS but no optic nerve damage
Primary angle-closure glaucoma (PACG)	Narrow angle with elevated IOP or PAS with evidence of optic nerve damage
Primary angle closure without pupillary block (plateau iris)	An anatomical variation in the iris root in which narrowing of the angle occurs independent of pupillary block
Chronic angle closure	IOP elevation caused by variable portions of anterior chamber angle being permanently closed by PAS
Secondary angle closure with pupillary block	Pupillary block occurs as a result of a mechanism other than the anatomical configuration of the anterior segment (eg, intumescent lens, air/gas/silicone oil bubble, secluded pupil, or DSAEK)
Secondary angle closure without pupillary block	Posterior pushing mechanism: lens–iris interface pushed forward (eg, posterior segment tumor, malignant glaucoma, uveal effusion, intravitreal injections)
	Anterior pulling mechanism: iris pulled forward to form PAS (eg, iridocorneal endothelial syndrome, neovascular glaucoma, inflammation)
Childhood glaucoma	
Primary congenital glaucoma (PCG)	Presents at birth or within the first few years of life
Glaucoma associated with congenital anomalies	Associated with ocular disorders (eg, Axenfeld-Rieger syndrome, aniridia)
	Associated with systemic disorders (eg, Sturge-Weber syndrome, neurofibromatosis 1)
Secondary glaucoma in infants and children	Associated with acquired disorders (eg, inflammation, retinoblastoma, trauma)

DSAEK = Descemet-stripping automated endothelial keratoplasty; IOP = intraocular pressure; PAS = peripheral anterior synechiae.

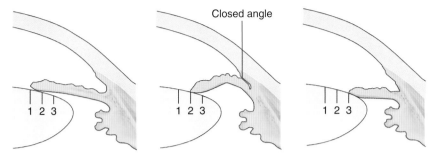

Figure 1-1 *1,* The pupil is constricted and the angle is open. *2,* The pupil is in the mid-dilated position. Pupillary block is maximal in this position and, as a result, the iris is bowed anteriorly and the angle narrows. *3,* The pupil is completely dilated, and pupillary block is diminished, with a return to a flatter iris configuration. If full-blown angle closure occurs, the iris may stay in the mid-dilated position until the angle-closure attack is broken. *(Illustration by Cyndie C. H. Wooley.)*

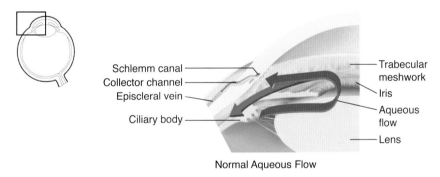

Figure 1-2 Diagrammatic cross section of the anterior segment of the normal eye, showing the site of aqueous production (ciliary body), sites of conventional aqueous outflow (trabecular meshwork–Schlemm canal system and episcleral venous plexus; *red arrow*), and the uveo-scleral outflow pathway *(green arrow). (Illustration by Cyndie C. H. Wooley.)*

there is no identifiable underlying anatomical cause of the events that led to obstruction of aqueous outflow and subsequent elevation of IOP. The etiology of the outflow obstruction is generally thought to be an abnormality in the extracellular matrix of the trabecular meshwork and in trabecular cells in the juxtacanalicular region, but other etiologies have been suggested. Glaucoma is classified as secondary when an abnormality is identified and a putative role in the pathogenesis of the disease can be ascribed to the abnormality. There are other approaches for classifying the glaucomas (eg, anatomical, gonioscopic, biochemical, molecular, and genetic), and each has its merit.

As knowledge of the mechanisms underlying the causes of glaucoma has grown, other schemes for classifying this disease have been proposed and the primary/secondary classification has become increasingly artificial. Classification of the glaucomas based on initial events and classification based on mechanisms of outflow obstruction are 2 schemes that have gained increasing popularity (Table 1-2).

Casson RJ, Chidlow G, Wood JP, Crowston JG, Goldberg I. Definition of glaucoma: clinical and experimental concepts. *Clin Experiment Ophthalmol.* 2012;40(4):341–349.

Table 1-2 Classification of the Glaucomas Based on Mechanisms of Outflow Obstruction*

Open-Angle Glaucoma Mechanisms			Angle-Closure Glaucoma Mechanisms		Developmental Anomalies of
Pretrabecular (Membrane Overgrowth)	Trabecular	Posttrabecular	Anterior ("Pulling")	Posterior ("Pushing")	Anterior Chamber Angle
Fibrovascular membrane (neovascular glaucoma)	Idiopathic	Obstruction of Schlemm canal, eg, collapse at canal	Contracture of membranes	**With pupillary block**	Incomplete development of trabecular meshwork–Schlemm canal and iris
Endothelial layer, often with Descemet-like membrane	Primary open-angle glaucoma	Elevated episcleral venous pressure	Neovascular glaucoma	Primary pupillary block glaucoma	Congenital (infantile) glaucoma
Iridocorneal endothelial syndrome	Juvenile open-angle glaucoma	Carotid-cavernous fistula	Iridocorneal endothelial syndrome	Lens-induced mechanisms	Anterior segment dysgenesis
Posterior polymorphous dystrophy	"Clogging" of trabecular meshwork	Cavernous sinus thrombosis	Posterior polymorphous dystrophy	Phacomorphic lens	Axenfeld-Rieger syndrome
Penetrating and nonpenetrating trauma	Red blood cells	Retrobulbar tumors	Penetrating and nonpenetrating trauma	Ectopia lentis	Peters anomaly
Epithelial downgrowth	Hemorrhagic glaucoma	Thyroid eye disease	Consolidation of inflammatory products	Aphakic vitreous or silicone oil block	Aniridia
Fibrous ingrowth	Ghost cell glaucoma	Superior vena cava obstruction		Posterior synechiae	Glaucomas associated with other developmental anomalies
Inflammatory membrane	Sickled red blood cells	Mediastinal tumors		Pseudophakia (esp. with ACIOL)	
Fuchs heterochromic uveitis	Macrophages	Sturge-Weber syndrome		Uveitis with iris bombé	
Luetic interstitial keratitis	Hemolytic glaucoma	Familial episcleral venous pressure elevation		**Without pupillary block**	
	Phacolytic glaucoma			Ciliary block (malignant) glaucoma	
	Melanomalytic glaucoma			Lens-induced mechanisms	
	Neoplastic cells			Phacomorphic lens	
	Primary ocular tumors			Ectopia lentis	
	Neoplastic tumors			Following lens extraction (forward vitreous shift)	
	Juvenile xanthogranuloma			Anterior rotation of ciliary body	
	Pigment particles			Uveal effusion	
	Pigmentary glaucoma			Central retinal vein occlusion	
	Pseudoexfoliation syndrome (glaucoma capsulare)			Panretinal photocoagulation	
	Melanoma			Scleral buckling	
	Protein			Annular choroidal detachment	
	Uveitis			Intraocular tumors	
	Lens-induced glaucoma			Melanoma	
	Viscoelastic agents			Retinoblastoma	
	Alterations of the trabecular meshwork			Cysts of the iris and ciliary body	
	Steroid-induced glaucoma			Persistent fetal vasculature	
	Edema/inflammation			Retinopathy of prematurity	
	Uveitis (trabeculitis)			Plateau iris syndrome	
	Scleritis and episcleritis				
	Alkali burns				
	Trauma (angle recession)				
	Laser trabeculoplasty				
	Intraocular foreign bodies (hemosiderosis, chalcosis)				

ACIOL = anterior chamber intraocular lens.

*Clinical examples cited in this table do not represent an inclusive list of the glaucomas.

Combined-Mechanism Glaucoma

In combined-mechanism glaucoma, most commonly, the patient has undergone success-ful treatment for a narrow angle but continues to demonstrate reduced outflow facility and elevated IOP in the absence of peripheral anterior synechiae. Less commonly, second-ary angle closure develops from other causes in a patient who has OAG. In this condition, IOP elevation can occur as a result of the following:

- the intrinsic resistance of the trabecular meshwork to aqueous outflow in OAG
- the direct anatomical obstruction of the filtering meshwork by synechiae in angle-closure glaucoma

Epidemiologic Aspects of Glaucoma

Primary Open-Angle Glaucoma

Magnitude of the problem

Primary open-angle glaucoma (POAG) poses a significant public health problem. In the United States, the estimated prevalence of POAG in individuals older than 40 years is 1.86% (95% confidence interval, 1.75%–1.96%), based on a meta-analysis of population-based studies. Applied to data from the 2000 US census, this percentage translates to nearly 2.22 million Americans affected. Estimates based on the available data indicate that between 84,000 and 116,000 of these individuals have become bilaterally blind (best-corrected visual acuity ≤20/200 or visual field <20°). With the rapidly aging US popu-lation, the number of POAG patients is estimated to increase by 50%, to 3.36 million, by 2020.

The World Health Organization (WHO) undertook an analysis of the literature to estimate the prevalence, incidence, and severity of the different types of glaucoma on a worldwide basis. Using data collected predominantly in the late 1980s and early 1990s, the WHO estimated the global population of persons with high IOP (>21 mm Hg) to be 104.5 million. The incidence of POAG was estimated at 2.4 million persons per year. Blindness prevalence for all types of glaucoma was estimated at more than 8 million per-sons, with 4 million cases caused by POAG. Glaucoma was theoretically calculated to ac-count for 12.3% of cases of blindness; it is therefore the second leading cause of blindness worldwide, following cataract.

Prevalence

The estimated prevalence (the total number of individuals with a disease at a specific time) of POAG varies widely across population-based samples. For example, the Rotterdam Study (northern European population) shows a prevalence of 0.8%, while the Barbados Eye Study (Caribbean population) shows a prevalence of 7% in individuals older than 40 years. In both of these studies, however, there is a significant increase in the prevalence of POAG in older individuals, with estimates for persons in their 70s being generally 3 to 8 times higher than estimates for persons in their 40s. Also, multiple population-based surveys have demonstrated a higher prevalence of POAG in specific ethnic groups. Among white persons aged 40 years and older, a prevalence of between 1.1% and 2.1% has been reported. The prevalence among black persons and Latino persons is up to 4 times higher compared with that among whites. Black individuals are also at greater risk of blindness due to POAG, and this risk increases with age: in persons aged 46–65 years, the likelihood of blindness due to POAG is 15 times higher among blacks than it is among whites.

Friedman DS, Wolfs RC, O'Colmain BJ, et al. Prevalence of open-angle glaucoma among adults in the United States. *Arch Ophthalmol.* 2004;122(4):532–538.

Javitt JC, McBean AM, Nicholson GA, Babish JD, Warren JL, Krakauer H. Undertreatment of glaucoma among black Americans. *N Engl J Med.* 1991;325:1418–1422.

Varma R, Ying Lai M, Francis BA, et al; Los Angeles Latino Eye Study Group. Prevalence of open-angle glaucoma and ocular hypertension in Latinos: the Los Angeles Latino Eye Study. *Ophthalmology.* 2004;111(8):1439–1448.

Incidence

The incidence (the number of new cases of a disease that develop during a specific period) of POAG has not been examined as much as the prevalence of POAG in population-based studies, and it varies widely. The Barbados Eye Study demonstrated, in a predominantly black population, a 4-year incidence of 2.2% in subjects older than 40 years. A much lower incidence was demonstrated in the Visual Impairment Project (based in Melbourne, Australia), which found a 5-year incidence of 1.1% for definite and probable POAG. Similarly, the Rotterdam Study found a 5-year incidence of 1.8% for definite and probable POAG. The Rochester Epidemiology Project found an annual incidence of 14.5 cases per 100,000 population (equivalent to a 5-year incidence of 0.72%) in Olmsted County, Minnesota.

Risk factors

In prospective studies, a number of risk factors have been found to be associated with progression of POAG. They include elevated IOP, reduced perfusion pressure, advanced age, positive family history, thin central corneas, and race/ethnicity (Table 1-3). The role of gender and of various systemic factors (eg, diabetes mellitus, hypertension, atherosclerotic and ischemic vascular diseases) in the development of glaucoma has been widely debated, and currently available data are inconclusive.

In the assessment of elevated IOP, the clinician should keep in mind circadian variation in IOP, the importance of which is increasingly being recognized. Current evidence, obtained under sleep laboratory conditions, suggests that in most subjects, peak IOP occurs in the early-morning hours and is therefore not seen in the routine clinical setting.

Dueker DK, Singh K, Lin SC, et al. Corneal thickness measurement in the management of primary open-angle glaucoma: a report by the American Academy of Ophthalmology. *Ophthalmology.* 2007;114(9):1779–1787.

Leske MC, Connell AM, Wu SY, et al. Incidence of open-angle glaucoma: the Barbados Eye Studies. The Barbados Eye Studies Group. *Arch Ophthalmol.* 2001;119(1):89–95.

Leske MC, Heijl A, Hyman L, et al. Predictors of long-term progression in the early manifest glaucoma trial. *Ophthalmology.* 2007;114(11):1965–1972.

Table 1-3 Risk Factors for Glaucomatous Progression

Risk Factor	Prospective Study
Increasing age	AGIS, CIGTS, EGPS, EMGT, OHTS
African ancestry	AGIS, CIGTS, CNTGS, OHTS (univariate)
Visual field severity	AGIS, EGPS, EMGT, OHTS
Diabetes mellitus	AGIS, OHTS (protective)
Disc hemorrhage	CNTGS, EMGT
Follow-up IOP	CNTGS, EMGT
Cup–disc ratio	EGPS, OHTS
Central corneal thickness	EGPS, OHTS
Pseudoexfoliation	EMGT
Initial IOP	EMGT
Female sex	CNTGS
Male sex	AGIS
Perfusion pressure	BES, LALES
Hispanic ethnicity	LALES

AGIS = Advanced Glaucoma Intervention Study; BES = Barbados Eye Study; CIGTS = Collaborative Initial Glaucoma Treatment Study; CNTGS = Collaborative Normal-Tension Glaucoma Study; EGPS = European Glaucoma Prevention Study; EMGT = Early Manifest Glaucoma Trial; LALES = Los Angeles Latino Eye Study; OHTS = Ocular Hypertension Treatment Study.

Primary Angle-Closure Glaucoma

Prevalence

The prevalence of primary angle-closure glaucoma (PACG) varies among different racial and ethnic groups. Among white populations in the United States and Europe, it is estimated at 0.1%. The prevalence in Inuit populations from the Arctic regions is 20 to 40 times higher than that in white populations and is the highest known. Estimates for Asian populations vary widely, but available data suggest that the prevalence of PACG in most Asian population groups is between the prevalence in whites and in the Inuit. Some studies have suggested that the prevalence of PACG among blacks is similar to that among whites; most cases of PACG in black patients are chronic.

Risk factors

The prevalence of PACG varies by sex as well as by race and ethnicity. Several population-based surveys show that women are at increased risk of PACG. Studies of normal eyes have shown that women have shallower anterior chambers than men. Older age is another risk factor. The depth and volume of the anterior chamber decrease with age, predisposing the eye to pupillary block. The prevalence of PACG with pupillary block thus increases with age. Acute PACG is most common between the ages of 55 and 65 years, but it can occur in young adults and has been reported in children. Although PACG may occur in eyes with any type of refractive error, the shallower anterior chamber depth of hyperopic eyes may predispose them to this disease. Plateau iris may be suspected when PACG is seen in myopic eyes. A positive family history of PACG may also increase the risk of this disease.

Cho HK, Kee C. Population-based glaucoma prevalence studies in Asians. *Surv Ophthalmol.* 2014;59(4):434–447.

Epstein DL, Allingham RR, Schuman JS, eds. *Chandler and Grant's Glaucoma.* 4th ed. Baltimore: Williams & Wilkins; 1997:641–646.

Ritch RM, Shields MB, Krupin T, eds. *The Glaucomas.* 2nd ed. St Louis: Mosby; 1996:753–765.

Genetics, Environmental Factors, and Glaucoma

The precise mechanism of inheritance of glaucoma is not clear. Many cases appear to have an autosomal dominant inheritance pattern that may be polygenic; the age of onset is late or variable; they demonstrate incomplete penetrance; and they may be substantially influenced by environmental factors. (See BCSC Section 2, *Fundamentals and Principles of Ophthalmology,* Part III, Genetics, for detailed discussion of inheritance patterns.) A positive family history is a risk factor for the development of POAG. The prevalence of glaucoma among siblings of glaucoma patients is approximately 10%.

The first gene described for POAG, *GLC1A* (also called the trabecular meshwork inducible glucocorticoid response/myocilin gene *[TIGR/MYOC]*), codes for the TIGR protein and is a trabecular meshwork glucocorticoid gene, located on chromosome 1. Mutations in *GLC1A* are present in 3% of the general OAG population. Additional OAG genes have been mapped, and many potential OAG genes are being explored. The percentage of genes known to be associated with specific types of glaucoma is small, largely because of the complex nature of the disease and because of the complicated interactions between multiple genetic loci and environmental factors (Table 1-4). Researchers are increasingly applying genomewide scanning techniques in large cohorts of glaucoma subjects. These techniques may be useful for determining which regions of the genome are associated with glaucoma.

Allingham RR, Liu Y, Rhee DJ. The genetics of primary open-angle glaucoma: a review. *Exp Eye Res.* 2009;88(4):837–844.

Stone EM, Fingert JH, Alward WL, et al. Identification of a gene that causes primary open angle glaucoma. *Science.* 1997;275(5300):668–670.

Wolfs RC, Klaver CC, Ramrattan RS, van Duijn CM, Hofman A, de Jong PT. Genetic risk of primary open-angle glaucoma: population-based familial aggregation study. *Arch Ophthalmol.* 1998;116(12):1640–1645.

Environmental Factors

Evidence that environmental factors can play a role in the etiology of glaucoma arises from studies of twins and from analysis of the season of birth of glaucoma patients. If glaucoma were genetically determined, identical twins would theoretically share this trait more often than would fraternal twins. In the Finnish Twin Cohort Study, 3 of 29 monozygotic twin pairs were concordant for POAG, compared with 1 of 79 dizygotic twin pairs. Although a higher percentage of monozygotic twins was concordant for glaucoma, most of these twin pairs were not. These data suggest that while genetic factors contribute to the etiology of glaucoma, other factors, such as environmental influences, are important.

Table 1-4 Currently Mapped Glaucoma Genes

Locus	Chromosome Location	Phenotype	Inheritance Pattern	Gene
GLC1A	1q23	JOAG and adult POAG	Dominant	TIGR/MYOC
GLC1B	2cen-q13	NTG, adult POAG	Dominant	—
GLC1C	3q21-24	Adult POAG	Dominant	—
GLC1D	8q23	Adult POAG	Dominant	—
GLC1E	10P15-14	NTG, adult POAG	Dominant	OPTN
GLC1F	7q35	Adult POAG	Dominant	—
GLC1G	5q22	Adult POAG	Dominant, complex	WDR36
GLC1I	15q11-q13	Adult POAG	Complex	—
GLC1J	9q22	Early POAG	Dominant	—
GLC1K	20p12	Early POAG	Dominant	—
GPDS1	7q35-q36	PDS	Dominant	—
GLC3A	2p21	Congenital	Recessive	CYP1B1
GLC3B	1p36	Congenital	Recessive	—
GLC3C	14q24.3	Congenital	Recessive	—
GLC3D	14q24.3	Congenital	Recessive	—
NNO1	11p	Nanophthalmos	Dominant	—
VMD2	11q12	Nanophthalmos	Dominant	—
MFRP	11q23	Nanophthalmos	Recessive	—
RIEG1	4q25	Rieger syndrome	Dominant	PITX2
RIEG2	13q14	Rieger syndrome	Dominant	—
IRID1	6p25	Iridogoniodysgenesis	Dominant	FOXC1
	7q35	PDS	Dominant	—
NPS	9q34	Nail-patella syndrome	Dominant	LMX1B
	15q24	PXE		LOXL1

JOAG = juvenile open-angle glaucoma; NTG = normal-tension glaucoma; PDS = pigment dispersion syndrome; POAG = primary open-angle glaucoma; PXE = pseudoexfoliation.

Genetic Testing

In the future, the management of some glaucoma patients will involve testing of multiple, and potentially interacting, genetic loci. Rapid advances in genetic techniques allowing this type of testing have been made. Advances in the study of genetic diseases, however, require accurate categorization of individuals and families with specific phenotypes. By appropriately identifying families with strong histories of glaucoma, the practicing ophthalmologist has an opportunity to provide important information to researchers in genetics. The cooperation of the clinician is thus critical to the advancement of this vital area of research.

CHAPTER 2

Intraocular Pressure and Aqueous Humor Dynamics

An understanding of *aqueous humor dynamics* is essential for the evaluation and management of glaucoma. As shown in Figure 1-2 in Chapter 1, aqueous humor (aqueous) is produced in the posterior chamber and flows through the pupil into the anterior chamber. Aqueous humor exits the eye by passing through the *trabecular meshwork* and into the *Schlemm canal* before draining into the venous system through a plexus of collector channels. Some aqueous exits the eye via the uveoscleral pathway, which is proposed to pass through the root of the iris and the ciliary body face, into the suprachoroidal space. The proportion of aqueous flowing through the trabecular pathway versus the uveoscleral pathway varies as a result of multiple factors. The modified *Goldmann equation* summarizes the relationship between many of these factors and the intraocular pressure (IOP) in the undisturbed eye:

$$P_0 = (F - U)/C + P_v$$

where P_0 is the IOP in mm Hg, F is the rate of aqueous formation in microliters per minute (µL/min), U is the rate of aqueous humor drainage through the pressure-insensitive uveoscleral pathway in microliters per minute (µL/min), C is the facility of outflow through the pressure-sensitive trabecular pathway in microliters per minute per mm Hg (µL/min/mm Hg), and P_v is the episcleral venous pressure in mm Hg. Resistance to outflow *(R)* is the inverse of facility *(C)*. Figure 2-1 illustrates the impact of reduced outflow facility *(C* value) of aqueous humor on IOP.

Aqueous Humor Production and Composition

Aqueous humor is produced by the ciliary processes at an average rate of 2–3 µL/min. The ciliary body contains about 80 ciliary processes, each of which is composed of a double layer of epithelium over a core of stroma and a rich supply of fenestrated capillaries (Fig 2-2). These capillaries are supplied mainly by branches of the major arterial circle of the iris. The apical surfaces of the outer pigmented and inner nonpigmented epithelial cell layers face each other. The nonpigmented epithelial cells are joined by tight junctions, which are an important component of the blood–aqueous barrier. The inner nonpigmented epithelial cells, which protrude into the posterior chamber, contain numerous

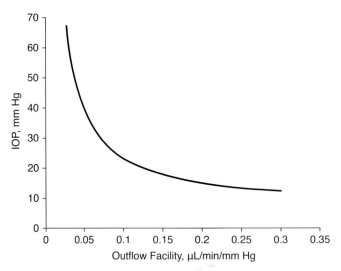

Figure 2-1 The effect of outflow facility on intraocular pressure (IOP), based on the modified Goldmann equation (assuming a constant aqueous humor production rate of 2.5 μL/min, uveoscleral outflow rate of 35%, and episcleral venous pressure of 7 mm Hg). *(Courtesy of Arthur J. Sit, MD.)*

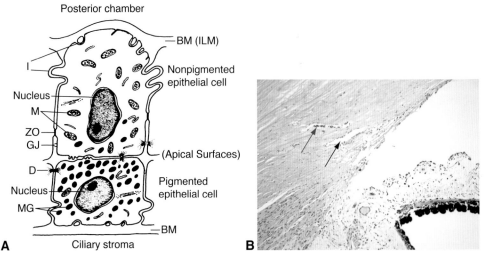

Figure 2-2 **A,** The 2 layers of the ciliary epithelium, showing apical surfaces in apposition to each other. Basement membrane (BM) lines the double layer and constitutes the internal limiting membrane (ILM) on the inner surface. The nonpigmented epithelium is characterized by large numbers of mitochondria (M), zonula occludens (ZO), and lateral and surface interdigitations (I). The pigmented epithelium contains numerous melanin granules (MG). Additional intercellular junctions include desmosomes (D) and gap junctions (GJ). **B,** Light micrograph of the anterior chamber angle shows the Schlemm canal *(black arrow),* adjacent to the trabecular meshwork in the sclera. One of the external collector vessels can be seen *(red arrow)* adjacent to the Schlemm canal.

(Continued)

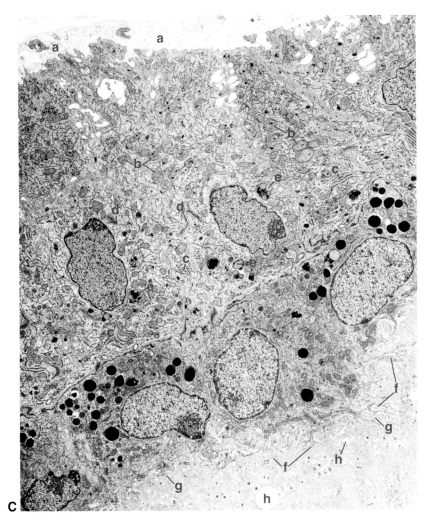

Figure 2-2 *(continued)* **C,** Pars plicata of the ciliary body showing the 2 epithelial layers in the eye of an older person. The nonpigmented epithelial cells measure approximately 20-μm high by 12-μm wide. The cuboidal pigmented epithelial cells are approximately 10-μm high. The thickened ILM *(a)* is laminated and vesicular; such thickened membranes are a characteristic of older eyes. The cytoplasm of the nonpigmented epithelium is characterized by its numerous mitochondria *(b)* and the cisternae of the rough-surfaced endoplasmic reticulum *(c)*. A poorly developed Golgi apparatus *(d)* and several lysosomes and residual bodies *(e)* are shown. The pigmented epithelium contains many melanin granules, measuring about 1 μm in diameter and located mainly in the apical portion. The basal surface is rather irregular, having many fingerlike processes *(f)*. The basement membrane of the pigmented epithelium *(g)* and a smooth granular material containing vesicles *(h)* and coarse granular particles are seen at the bottom of the figure. The appearance of the basement membrane is typical of older eyes and can be discerned with the light microscope (×5700). *(Part A reproduced with permission from Shields MB.* Textbook of Glaucoma. *3rd ed. Baltimore: Williams & Wilkins; 1992. Part B courtesy of Nasreen A. Syed, MD. Part C modified with permission from Hogan MJ, Alvarado JA, Weddell JE.* Histology of the Human Eye. *Philadelphia: Saunders; 1971:283.)*

mitochondria and microvilli; these cells are thought to be the actual site of aqueous production. The ciliary processes provide a large surface area for secretion.

Aqueous humor enters the posterior chamber via the following physiologic mechanisms:

- active secretion, which takes place in the double-layered ciliary epithelium
- ultrafiltration
- simple diffusion

Active secretion refers to transport that requires energy to move sodium, chloride, bicarbonate, and other ions, which are currently unknown, against an electrochemical gradient. Active secretion is independent of pressure and accounts for the majority of aqueous production. It involves, at least in part, activity of the enzyme carbonic anhydrase II. *Ultrafiltration* refers to a pressure-dependent movement along a pressure gradient. In the ciliary processes, the hydrostatic pressure difference between capillary pressure and IOP favors fluid movement into the eye, whereas the oncotic gradient between the two resists fluid movement. The relationship between secretion and ultrafiltration is not known. *Diffusion* involves the passive movement of ions, based on charge and concentration, across a membrane.

In humans, aqueous humor has an excess of hydrogen and chloride ions, an excess of ascorbate, and a deficit of bicarbonate relative to plasma. Aqueous humor is essentially protein free (1/200–1/500 of the protein found in plasma), allowing for optical clarity and reflecting the integrity of the blood–aqueous barrier of the normal eye. Albumin accounts for approximately half of the total protein. Other components of aqueous humor include growth factors; several enzymes, such as carbonic anhydrase, lysozyme, diamine oxidase, plasminogen activator, dopamine β-hydroxylase, and phospholipase A_2; and prostaglandins, cyclic adenosine monophosphate, catecholamines, steroid hormones, and hyaluronic acid. Aqueous humor composition is altered as it flows from the posterior chamber, through the pupil, and into the anterior chamber. This alteration occurs across the hyaloid face of the vitreous, the surface of the lens, the blood vessels of the iris, and the corneal endothelium; and it is secondary to other dilutional exchanges and active processes. See BCSC Section 2, *Fundamentals and Principles of Ophthalmology,* for further discussion of aqueous humor composition and production.

Suppression of Aqueous Formation

Various classes of drugs can suppress aqueous formation. The mechanisms of action of these drugs are discussed in Chapter 7.

Inhibition of the enzyme carbonic anhydrase suppresses aqueous humor formation. However, the precise role of carbonic anhydrase has been debated vigorously. Its function may be to provide the bicarbonate ion, which, evidence suggests, is actively secreted in human eyes. Carbonic anhydrase may also provide bicarbonate or hydrogen ions for an intracellular buffering system.

Aqueous humor formation may be reduced by the blockade of β_2-receptors, which are the most prevalent adrenergic receptors in the ciliary epithelium and which may affect active secretion by causing a decrease either in the efficiency of Na^+,K^+-ATPase or in the number of pump sites. For additional discussion of the sodium pump and the pump–leak mechanism, see BCSC Section 2, *Fundamentals and Principles of Ophthalmology*. Stimulation of α_2-receptors also reduces aqueous humor formation, possibly via a reduction of ciliary body blood flow mediated through inhibition of cyclic adenosine monophosphate (cAMP); the exact mechanism is unclear.

Measurement of Aqueous Formation

The most common method used to measure the rate of aqueous formation is *fluorophotometry*. For this test, fluorescein is administered systemically or topically, its gradual dilution in the anterior chamber is measured optically, and change in fluorescein concentration over time is then used to calculate aqueous flow. As previously noted, the normal flow is approximately 2–3 μL/min, and the aqueous volume is turned over at a rate of approximately 1% per minute. The measurement of aqueous humor flow rate is assumed to be equal to the rate of aqueous production by the ciliary processes at steady state.

The rate of aqueous humor formation varies diurnally and decreases by half during sleep. It also decreases with age. The rate of aqueous formation is affected by a variety of factors, including the following:

- integrity of the blood–aqueous barrier
- blood flow to the ciliary body
- neurohumoral regulation of vascular tissue and the ciliary epithelium

Aqueous humor production may decrease after trauma or intraocular inflammation and after the administration of certain drugs (eg, general anesthetics and some systemic hypotensive agents). Carotid occlusive disease may also decrease aqueous humor production.

Brubaker RF. Flow of aqueous humor in humans [The Friedenwald Lecture]. *Invest Ophthalmol Vis Sci.* 1991;32(13):3145–3166.

Aqueous Humor Outflow

Aqueous humor outflow occurs by 2 major mechanisms: pressure-sensitive trabecular outflow and pressure-insensitive uveoscleral outflow.

Trabecular Outflow

The trabecular meshwork is classically divided into 3 layers: uveal, corneoscleral, and juxtacanalicular (Fig 2-3). The *uveal trabecular meshwork* is adjacent to the anterior chamber and is arranged in bands that extend from the iris root and the ciliary body to the peripheral cornea. The *corneoscleral meshwork* consists of sheets of trabeculum that extend from the scleral spur to the lateral wall of the scleral sulcus. The *juxtacanalicular meshwork,* which is thought to be the major site of outflow resistance, is adjacent to and actually forms the inner wall of the Schlemm canal. Aqueous moves both across and between the endothelial cells lining the inner wall of the Schlemm canal.

The trabecular meshwork is composed of multiple layers, each of which consists of a collagenous connective tissue core covered by a continuous endothelial layer. The trabecular meshwork is the site of pressure-sensitive outflow and functions as a one-way valve,

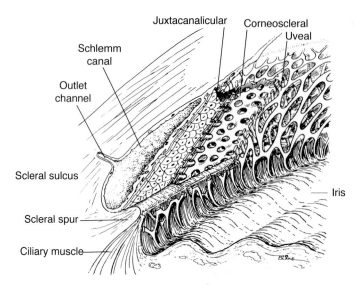

Juxtacanalicular   Corneoscleral
Uveal
Schlemm
canal
Outlet
channel
Scleral sulcus
Iris
Scleral spur
Ciliary muscle

Figure 2-3 Three layers of the trabecular meshwork *(shown in cutaway views):* uveal, corneo-scleral, and juxtacanalicular. *(Modified with permission from Shields MB.* Textbook of Glaucoma. *3rd ed. Baltimore: Williams & Wilkins; 1992.)*

permitting aqueous to leave the eye by bulk flow but limiting flow in the other direction, independent of energy. Its cells are phagocytic, and they may exhibit this function in the presence of inflammation and after laser trabeculoplasty.

In most eyes of older adults, trabecular cells contain a large number of pigment granules within their cytoplasm that give the entire meshwork a brown or muddy appearance. There are relatively few trabecular cells—approximately 200,000–300,000 cells per eye. With age, the number of trabecular cells decreases, and the basement membrane beneath them thickens, potentially increasing outflow resistance. An interesting effect of all types of laser trabeculoplasty is that it induces division of trabecular cells and causes a change in the production of cytokines and other structurally important elements of the extracellular matrix. The extracellular matrix material is found through the dense portions of the trabecular meshwork.

The *Schlemm canal* is completely lined with an endothelial layer that rests on a discontinuous basement membrane. The canal is a single channel, typically with a diameter of about 200–300 μm, although there is significant variability; it is traversed by tubules. The exact path of aqueous flow across the inner wall of the Schlemm canal is uncertain. Intracellular and intercellular pores suggest bulk flow, while so-called giant vacuoles that have direct communication with the intertrabecular spaces suggest active transport but may be artifacts. The outer wall of the Schlemm canal is formed by a single layer of endothelial cells that do not contain pores. A complex system of vessels connects the Schlemm canal to the episcleral veins, which subsequently drain into the anterior ciliary and superior ophthalmic veins. These, in turn, ultimately drain into the cavernous sinus.

The trabecular outflow pathway is dynamic. With increasing IOP, the cross-sectional area of the Schlemm canal decreases, while the trabecular meshwork expands. The effect of these changes on outflow resistance is unclear.

Measurement of Outflow Facility

The facility of outflow (C in the Goldmann equation; see the beginning of the chapter) is the mathematical inverse of outflow resistance and varies widely in normal eyes, with mean value ranging from 0.22 to 0.30 μL/min/mm Hg. Outflow facility decreases with age and is affected by surgery, trauma, medications, and endocrine factors. Patients with glaucoma and elevated IOP typically have decreased outflow facility.

Tonography is a method used to measure the facility of aqueous outflow. With this technique, a weighted Schiøtz tonometer or pneumatonometer is placed on the cornea, acutely elevating the IOP. Outflow facility in μL/min/mm Hg can be computed from the rate at which the pressure declines with time, reflecting the ease with which aqueous leaves the eye.

Unfortunately, tonography depends on a number of assumptions (eg, ocular rigidity, stability of aqueous formation, and constancy of ocular blood volume) and is subject to many sources of error, such as patient fixation and eyelid squeezing. These problems reduce the accuracy and reproducibility of tonography for an individual patient. In general, tonography is best used as a research tool for investigating mechanisms of action of IOP changes and is rarely used clinically.

Uveoscleral Outflow

In the normal eye, any nontrabecular outflow is termed *uveoscleral outflow.* Uveoscleral outflow is also referred to as *pressure-insensitive outflow.* A variety of mechanisms are likely involved, but the predominant one is aqueous passage from the anterior chamber into the ciliary muscle and then into the supraciliary and suprachoroidal spaces. The fluid then exits the eye through the intact sclera or along the nerves and the vessels that penetrate it. There is evidence that outflow via the uveoscleral pathway is significant in human eyes, accounting for up to 45% of total aqueous outflow. Studies indicate that uveoscleral outflow decreases with age and is reduced in patients with glaucoma. It is increased by cycloplegia, adrenergic agents, and prostaglandin analogues but decreased by miotics. It is also increased by certain complications of surgery and by cyclodialysis clefts. Uveoscleral outflow cannot be measured noninvasively and is therefore calculated from the Goldmann equation.

Brubaker RF. Measurement of uveoscleral outflow in humans. *J Glaucoma.* 2001;10(5 Suppl 1): S45–S48.

Johnson M. 'What controls aqueous humour outflow resistance?' *Exp Eye Res.* 2006;82(4): 545–557.

Episcleral Venous Pressure

Episcleral venous pressure (EVP) is relatively stable, except with alterations in body position and with certain diseases that obstruct venous return to the heart or shunt blood from the arterial to the venous system. Episcleral venous pressure is often increased in syndromes with facial hemangiomas (eg, Sturge-Weber), carotid-cavernous sinus fistulas, and cavernous sinus thrombosis, and it is partially responsible for the elevated IOP seen in thyroid eye disease. The pressure in the episcleral veins can be measured with specialized equipment. The usual range of values is 6–9 mm Hg, but higher values have been reported depending on the measurement technique used. According to the Goldmann equation, IOP rises approximately 1 mm Hg for every 1 mm Hg increase in EVP. However, elevation of EVP may alter other parameters of aqueous humor dynamics. Abnormally elevated EVP can cause collapse of the Schlemm canal and potentially increase aqueous humor outflow resistance; elevated EVP may also alter uveoscleral outflow. As a result, the change in IOP may be greater or less than that predicted by the Goldmann equation.

Sit AJ, McLaren JW. Measurement of episcleral venous pressure. *Exp Eye Res.* 2011;93(3): 291–298.

Intraocular Pressure

Distribution in the Population and Relation to Glaucoma

Pooled data from large epidemiologic studies indicate that the mean IOP in the general population of European ancestry is approximately 15.5 mm Hg, with a standard deviation of 2.6 mm Hg. However, IOP has a non-Gaussian distribution with a skew toward higher pressures, especially in individuals older than 40 years (Fig 2-4). The value 21 mm Hg (>2 standard deviations above the mean) was traditionally used both to separate normal and abnormal pressures and to define which patients required ocular hypotensive therapy. This division was based on 2 erroneous clinical assumptions, which are as follows: glaucomatous damage is caused exclusively by pressures that are higher than normal; and normal pressures do not cause damage. An example of the shortcomings created by these assumptions

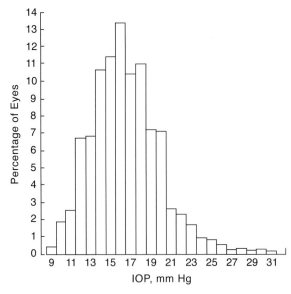

Figure 2-4 Frequency distribution of IOP: 5220 eyes in the Framingham Eye Study. *(Modified from Colton T, Ederer F. The distribution of intraocular pressures in the general population.* Surv Ophthalmol. *1980;25:123–129.)*

is that screening for glaucoma based solely on IOP greater than 21 mm Hg misses up to half of the people with glaucoma and optic nerve damage in the screened population.

General agreement has been reached that, for the population as a whole, there is no clear IOP level below which IOP can be considered "normal" or safe and above which IOP can be considered "elevated" or unsafe. In some eyes, damage occurs with IOP levels of 18 mm Hg or lower, whereas in other eyes, IOPs of 30 mm Hg or higher are tolerated. However, elevation of IOP is considered a very important risk factor for glaucoma. Although other risk factors affect an individual's susceptibility to glaucoma, all current treatments are designed to reduce IOP.

Factors Influencing Intraocular Pressure

Intraocular pressure varies with a number of factors, including the time of day (see the subsection "Circadian variation"), body position, heartbeat, respiration, exercise, fluid intake, systemic medications, and topical medications (Table 2-1). Also, IOP is genetically

Table 2-1 Factors That Affect Intraocular Pressure

Factors that may increase intraocular pressure
Elevated episcleral venous pressure
  Bending over or being in a supine position
  Breath holding
  Elevated central venous pressure
  Intubation
  Orbital venous outflow obstruction
  Playing a wind instrument
  Valsalva maneuver
  Wearing a tight collar or tight necktie
Pressure on the eye
  Blepharospasm
  Squeezing and crying, especially in young children
Elevated body temperature: associated with increased aqueous humor production
Hormonal influences
  Hypothyroidism
  Thyroid eye disease
Drugs unrelated to glaucoma therapy
  Anticholinergics: may precipitate angle closure
  Corticosteroids
  Ketamine
  Lysergic acid diethylamide (LSD)
  Topiramate

Factors that may decrease intraocular pressure
Aerobic exercise
Anesthetic drugs
  Depolarizing muscle relaxants such as succinylcholine
Metabolic or respiratory acidosis: decreases aqueous humor production
Hormonal influences
  Pregnancy
Drugs unrelated to glaucoma therapy
  Alcohol
  Heroin
  Marijuana (cannabis)

influenced: higher pressures are more common in relatives of patients with primary open-angle glaucoma than in the general population.

IOP is higher when an individual is recumbent rather than upright, predominantly because of an increase in the EVP. Some individuals have an exaggerated rise in IOP when recumbent; this tendency may be important in the pathogenesis of some forms of glaucoma. Alcohol consumption results in a transient decrease in IOP. In most studies, caffeine has not been shown to have an appreciable effect on IOP. Cannabis also decreases IOP but has not been proven clinically useful because of its short duration of action and poor side-effect profile. Finally, there is little variation in IOP with age in healthy individuals.

Circadian variation

In individuals without glaucoma, IOP varies by 2–6 mm Hg over a 24-hour period, as aqueous humor production, outflow facility, and uveoscleral outflow rate change. Higher IOP is associated with wider fluctuation in pressure. The time at which peak IOPs occur in any individual is quite variable. In many persons, peak daytime pressures are reached in the morning. However, around-the-clock IOP measurement performed with individuals in habitual body positions (standing or sitting during the daytime and supine at night) indicates that in most persons (those with glaucoma and those without) peak pressures are reached during sleep, in the early-morning hours. Measurement of IOP outside office hours may be useful for determining why optic nerve damage occurs despite apparently adequately controlled pressure. However, the impact of IOP fluctuations on the optic nerve remains unknown.

Liu JH, Zhang X, Kripke DF, Weinreb RN. Twenty-four-hour intraocular pressure pattern associated with early glaucomatous changes. *Invest Ophthalmol Vis Sci.* 2003;44(4): 1586–1590.

Nau CB, Malihi M, McLaren JW, Hodge DO, Sit AJ. Circadian variation of aqueous humor dynamics in older healthy adults. *Invest Ophthalmol Vis Sci.* 2013;54(12):7623–7629.

Clinical Measurement of Intraocular Pressure

Tonometry is the noninvasive measurement of IOP. *Applanation tonometry,* the most widely used method, is based on the Imbert-Fick principle, which states that the pressure inside an ideal dry, thin-walled sphere equals the force necessary to flatten its surface divided by the area of the flattening:

$$P = F/A$$

where P = pressure, F = force, and A = area. In applanation tonometry, the cornea is flattened, and IOP is determined by measuring the applanating force and the area flattened.

The *Goldmann applanation tonometer* (Fig 2-5) measures the force necessary to flatten an area of the cornea of 3.06 mm in diameter. At this diameter, the material resistance of the cornea to flattening is counterbalanced by the capillary attraction of the tear film meniscus to the tonometer head. Furthermore, the IOP (in mm Hg) equals the flattening force (in grams-force) multiplied by 10. A split-image prism allows the examiner to determine the flattened area with great accuracy. To outline the area of flattening, topical anesthetic and fluorescein dye are instilled in the tear film. Fluorescein semicircles, or

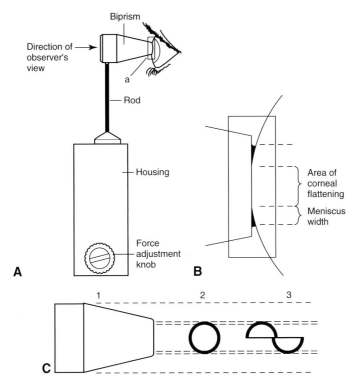

Figure 2-5 Goldmann-type applanation tonometry. **A,** Basic features of the tonometer, shown in contact with the patient's cornea. **B,** The enlargement shows the tear film meniscus created by contact of the split-image prism and cornea. **C,** The view through the split-image prism (1) reveals circular meniscus (2), which is converted into 2 semicircles (3) by the prisms. *(Redrawn with permission from Shields MB.* Textbook of Glaucoma. *3rd ed. Baltimore: Williams & Wilkins; 1992.)*

mires, visible through the split-image prism move with the ocular pulse, and the endpoint is reached when the inner edges of the semicircles touch each other at the midpoint of their excursion (Fig 2-6). By properly aligning the mires, the examiner can ensure the appropriate area of corneal applanation and obtain a correct IOP reading.

The *Perkins tonometer* is a counterbalanced applanation tonometer that, like the Goldmann tonometer, uses a split-image prism and requires instillation of fluorescein dye in the tear film. It is portable and can be used with the patient either upright or supine.

Applanation measurements are safe, easy to perform, and relatively accurate in most clinical situations. Of the currently available devices, the Goldmann applanation tonometer is the most widely used in clinical practice and for studies. Because applanation does not displace much fluid (approximately 0.5 µL) or substantially increase the pressure in the eye, IOP measurement by this method is relatively unaffected by ocular rigidity, compared with indentation tonometry.

The accuracy of applanation tonometry is reduced in certain situations, however (see Table 2-2, which lists possible sources of error in tonometry). For example, an excessive amount of fluorescein in the tear film results in wide mires and an artificially high reading, whereas an inadequate amount of fluorescein leads to artificially low readings. If

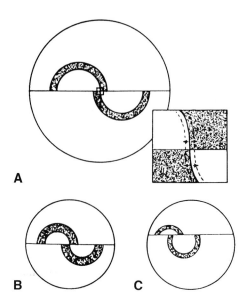

Figure 2-6 Mires viewed through the split-image prism of the Goldmann-type applanation tonometer. **A,** Proper width and position. The enlargement depicts excursions of the mires, which are caused by ocular pulsations. **B,** The mires are too wide. **C,** Improper vertical and horizontal alignment. *(Reproduced with permission from Shields MB.* Textbook of Glaucoma. *3rd ed. Baltimore: Williams & Wilkins; 1992.)*

Table 2-2 Possible Sources of Error in Tonometry

Factors that may cause artificially low IOP	Factors that may cause artificially high IOP
Corneal biomechanical properties (eg, rigidity)	Breath holding or Valsalva maneuver
Corneal edema	Corneal biomechanical properties (eg, rigidity)
Corneal irregularity (eg, ectasia)	Corneal irregularity (eg, ectasia)
High corneal astigmatism	Corneal scarring or band keratopathy
Inaccurately calibrated tonometer	Excessive amount of fluorescein in tear film
Inadequate amount of fluorescein in tear film	Extraocular muscle force applied to a restricted globe
Measurement done over a soft contact lens	High corneal astigmatism
Technician errors	Inaccurately calibrated tonometer
Thin central cornea	Obesity or straining to reach slit lamp
	Pressure on the globe
	Squeezing of the eyelids
	Technician errors
	Thick central cornea
	Tight collar or tight necktie

IOP = intraocular pressure.

the patient has marked corneal astigmatism, the fluorescein pattern seen by the clinician through the instrument ocular is elliptical and the IOP may be artificially high or low. To obtain an accurate reading, the clinician should rotate the prism so that the red mark on the prism holder is set at the least-curved meridian of the cornea (along the negative axis). Alternatively, 2 pressure readings taken 90° apart can be averaged. Corneal edema predisposes to falsely low readings, whereas pressure measurements taken over a corneal scar will be falsely high. Tonometry performed over a soft contact lens gives falsely low values. Central corneal thickness is another factor that can affect the accuracy of tonometry; see the following subsection.

Tonometry and central corneal thickness

Measurements obtained with the most common types of tonometers are affected by central corneal thickness (CCT). Measurement with the Goldmann tonometer is most accurate when the CCT is 520 μm. Thicker corneas resist the deformation inherent in most methods of tonometry, resulting in an overestimation of IOP, while thinner corneas may give an artificially low reading. IOP measured after photorefractive keratectomy and laser in situ keratomileusis may be underestimated because of changes in corneal thickness induced by these and other refractive procedures.

The relationship between measured IOP and CCT is not linear, so any correction factors are only estimates at best. In addition, the biomechanical properties of individual corneas may vary, and the stiffness or elasticity of the cornea may affect IOP measurement. Currently, there is no validated correction factor for the effect of CCT on applanation tonometers; therefore, clinical application of any of the correction methods proposed in the literature should be avoided. Thin CCT is a risk factor for progression from ocular hypertension to glaucoma, but whether this increased risk of glaucoma is due to underestimating actual IOP in patients with thin central corneas or whether a thin central cornea is a risk factor independent of IOP measurement has not been determined (see Chapter 4).

Brandt JD. The influence of corneal thickness on the diagnosis and management of glaucoma. *J Glaucoma.* 2001;10(5 Suppl 1):S65–S67.

Gordon MO, Beiser JA, Brandt JA, et al. The Ocular Hypertension Treatment Study: baseline factors that predict the onset of primary open-angle glaucoma. *Arch Ophthalmol.* 2002; 120(6):714–720.

Sommer A, Tielsch JM, Katz J, et al. Relationship between intraocular pressure and primary open-angle glaucoma among white and black Americans. The Baltimore Eye Survey. *Arch Ophthalmol.* 1991;109(8):1090–1095.

Methods other than Goldmann-type applanation tonometry

While applanation tonometry remains the standard clinical method for measurement of IOP, numerous other methods have been developed, each with advantages and disadvantages when compared with applanation.

Mackay-Marg-type tonometers use an annular ring to gently flatten a small area of the cornea. As the area of flattening increases, the pressure in the center of the ring increases as well and is measured with a transducer. The IOP is equivalent to the pressure when the center of the ring is just covered by the flattened cornea.

Portable electronic devices of the Mackay-Marg type (eg, Tono-Pen, Reichert Technologies, Depew, NY) contain a strain gauge to measure the pressure at the center of an annular ring placed on the cornea. These devices are particularly useful for measuring IOP in patients with corneal scars or edema.

The *pneumatic tonometer,* or *pneumatonometer,* is an applanation tonometer that shares some characteristics with the Mackay-Marg-type devices. It has a cylindrical air-filled chamber and a probe tip covered with a flexible, inert silicone elastomer (Silastic membrane) diaphragm. Because of the constant flow of air through the chamber, there is a small gap between the diaphragm and the probe edge. As the probe tip touches and applanates the cornea, the air pressure increases until this gap is completely closed, at which point the IOP is equivalent to the air pressure. Because this instrument covers only a small area of the cornea, it is especially useful in eyes with corneal scars or edema.

The *dynamic contour tonometer,* a newer type of nonapplanation contact tonometer, is based on the principle that when the surface of the cornea is aligned with the surface of the instrument tip, the pressure in the tear film between these surfaces is equal to the IOP and can be measured by a pressure transducer. Evidence suggests that IOP measurements obtained with dynamic contour tonometry are more independent of corneal biomechanical properties and thickness than those obtained with older tonometers.

Noncontact (air-puff) tonometers determine IOP by measuring the force of air required to indent the cornea to a fixed point, thereby avoiding contact with the eye. Readings obtained with these instruments vary widely, and IOP is often overestimated. Noncontact tonometers are often used in large-scale glaucoma-screening programs or by nonmedical health care providers.

The *Ocular Response Analyzer* (ORA; Reichert Technologies, Depew, NY) is a type of noncontact tonometer that uses correction algorithms so that its IOP readings more closely match applanation IOPs and the effect of corneal biomechanical properties on pressure measurement is reduced. In addition, indicators of ocular biomechanical properties are calculated, including corneal hysteresis and corneal resistance factor. Corneal hysteresis is the difference in IOP measured during the initial corneal indentation and IOP measured during corneal rebound. Reduced corneal hysteresis may be a risk factor for glaucoma.

Rebound tonometry determines IOP by measuring the speed at which a small probe propelled against the cornea decelerates and rebounds after impact. Rebound tonometers are portable, and topical anesthesia is not required, making them particularly suitable for pediatric populations. The current instrument should be used upright.

Schiøtz tonometry determines IOP by measuring the amount of corneal indentation produced by a known weight. The amount of indentation is read on a linear scale on the instrument and converted to mm Hg by a calibration table. Due to a number of practical and theoretical problems, Schiøtz tonometry is now rarely used in the developed world.

It is possible to estimate IOP by *digital pressure* on the globe, referred to as *tactile tension.* This test may be useful in uncooperative patients; however, the results may be inaccurate even when the test is performed by very experienced clinicians. In general, tactile tensions are useful only for detecting large differences in IOP between a patient's two eyes.

Durham DG, Bigliano RP, Masino JA. Pneumatic applanation tonometer. *Trans Am Acad Ophthalmol Otolaryngol.* 1965;69(6):1029–1047.

Kontiola AI. A new induction-based impact method for measuring intraocular pressure. *Acta Ophthalmol Scand.* 2000;78(2):142–145.

Luce DA. Determining in vivo biomechanical properties of the cornea with an ocular response analyzer. *J Cataract Refract Surg.* 2005;31(1):156–162.

Mackay RS, Marg E. Fast, automatic, electronic tonometers based on an exact theory. *Acta Ophthalmol (Copenh).* 1959;37:495–507.

Infection control in clinical tonometry

Many infectious agents—including the viruses responsible for acquired immunodeficiency syndrome, hepatitis, and epidemic keratoconjunctivitis—can be recovered from tears. Tonometers must be cleaned after each use so that the transfer of such agents can be prevented. For Goldmann-type tonometers and the Perkins tonometer, the tonometer tips (prisms) should be cleaned immediately after use. The prisms should be soaked in a 1:10 sodium hypochlorite solution (household bleach), in 3% hydrogen peroxide, or in 70% isopropyl alcohol for 5 minutes and rinsed and dried before reuse. If alcohol is employed, it should be allowed to evaporate or the prism head should be dried before reuse to prevent damage to the corneal epithelium. For cleaning other tonometers, refer to the manufacturer's recommendations.

CHAPTER 3

Clinical Evaluation

History and General Examination

Appropriate management of glaucoma depends on the clinician's ability to diagnose the specific form of glaucoma in a given patient, to determine the severity of the condition, to predict the likelihood of progression, and to detect progression when it occurs. Clinical evaluation of the glaucoma patient should include a history of the current complaint, including symptoms, onset, duration, and severity. Past ocular history (medical and surgical) and a general medical history, including the patient's current medications and allergies, should be obtained. On physical examination, prior to biomicroscopy, it is helpful to record the patient's pulse and blood pressure.

The clinician should inquire about symptoms often associated with glaucoma, such as pain, redness, colored halos around lights, alteration of vision, and loss of vision. Similarly, the general medical history should include specific inquiry about diseases or conditions that may have ocular manifestations or that may affect the patient's ability to tolerate medications. Such conditions include diabetes mellitus, cardiac and pulmonary disease, hypertension, hemodynamic shock, systemic hypotension, sleep apnea, Raynaud phenomenon, migraine and other neurologic diseases, renal stones, and pregnancy. The clinician should take note of a history of corticosteroid use, either topical or systemic. See also BCSC Section 1, *Update on General Medicine*.

Refraction

Neutralizing any refractive error is crucial for accurate perimetry with most perimeters, and the clinician should understand how the patient's refractive state could affect the diagnosis. The hyperopic eye is at increased risk of angle-closure and generally has a smaller optic nerve head (also called optic disc). Myopia is associated with optic nerve head morphologies that can be clinically confused with glaucoma, and myopic eyes are at increased risk of pigment dispersion.

External Adnexae

Examination and assessment of the external ocular adnexae is useful for determining the presence of a variety of conditions associated with secondary glaucomas as well as external ocular manifestations of glaucoma therapy. The entities described in this section are discussed in greater depth and illustrated in other volumes of the BCSC series; consult the *Master Index*.

An example of an association between adnexal changes and systemic disease is *tuberous sclerosis (Bourneville syndrome),* in which glaucoma may occur secondary to vitreous hemorrhage, anterior segment neovascularization, or retinal detachment. Typical external and cutaneous signs of tuberous sclerosis include a hypopigmented lesion termed the "ash-leaf sign" and a red-brown papular rash (adenoma sebaceum) that is often found on the face and chin.

Other changes in the ocular adnexa associated with secondary glaucoma include the subcutaneous plexiform neuromas that are a hallmark of the type 1 variant of neurofibromatosis, the yellow and/or orange papules in *juvenile xanthogranuloma,* and the skin pigmentation seen in *oculodermal melanocytosis (nevus of Ota).*

Several entities are associated with signs of elevated episcleral venous pressure (see the section Elevated Episcleral Venous Pressure in Chapter 4). The presence of a facial cutaneous angioma (nevus flammeus, or port-wine stain) can indicate *encephalofacial angiomatosis (Sturge-Weber syndrome).* Hemifacial hypertrophy may also be observed. The cutaneous hemangiomas of the *Klippel-Trénaunay-Weber syndrome* extend over an affected, secondarily hypertrophied limb and may also involve the face. Orbital varices, arteriovenous fistulas, and superior vena cava syndrome may also be associated with elevated episcleral venous pressure and secondary glaucoma. Intermittent unilateral proptosis and dilated eyelid veins are key external signs of *orbital varices. Carotid-cavernous, dural-cavernous,* and other *arteriovenous fistulas* can produce orbital bruits, restricted ocular motility, proptosis, and pulsating exophthalmos. *Superior vena cava syndrome* can cause proptosis and facial and eyelid edema, as well as conjunctival chemosis. *Thyroid eye disease* may also be associated with glaucoma; ophthalmic features of this disease include exophthalmos, eyelid retraction, and motility disorders.

Use of prostaglandin analogues may result in cosmetic changes to the ocular adnexa; these are described in Chapter 7.

Pupils

Pupil size may be affected by glaucoma therapy, and pupillary responses are one measure of adherence in patients who are on miotic therapy. Testing for a relative afferent pupillary defect may detect asymmetric optic nerve damage. Corectopia, ectropion uveae, and pupillary abnormalities may also be observed in some forms of secondary open-angle glaucoma and angle-closure glaucoma. In some clinical situations, it is not possible to assess the pupils objectively for the presence of a relative afferent defect, and a subjective comparison between the eyes of the perceived brightness of a test light may be helpful. Testing for color vision, extraocular motility, and cranial nerve abnormality can also be helpful in the differential diagnosis of nonglaucomatous versus glaucomatous optic neuropathy.

Biomicroscopy

Biomicroscopy of the anterior segment is performed for signs of underlying ocular conditions that may be associated with glaucoma. BCSC Section 8, *External Disease and Cornea,* discusses slit-lamp technique and the examination of the external eye in greater depth.

Conjunctiva

Eyes with acutely elevated intraocular pressure (IOP) may show conjunctival hyperemia. Long-term use of sympathomimetics and prostaglandin analogues may also cause conjunctival hyperemia, and long-term use of epinephrine derivatives may result in black adrenochrome deposits in the conjunctiva. Allergic reaction to ocular hypotensive medications (especially α_2-adrenergic agonists) may be accompanied by a follicular reaction. The use of topical ocular hypotensive medication can also cause decreased tear production, allergic and hypersensitivity reactions (papillary and follicular conjunctivitis), foreshortening of the conjunctival fornices, and scarring. Prior to filtering surgery, the presence or absence of subconjunctival scarring or other conjunctival abnormalities should be assessed. The presence or absence of any filtering bleb should be noted. If a bleb is present, its size, height, degree of vascularization, and integrity should be noted, and in the situation of postoperative hypotony, a Seidel test performed.

Episclera and sclera

Dilation of the episcleral vessels may indicate elevated episcleral venous pressure, as seen in the secondary glaucomas associated with Sturge-Weber syndrome, arteriovenous fistulae, or thyroid eye disease. Sentinel vessels may be seen in eyes harboring an intraocular tumor. The clinician should note any thinning or staphylomatous areas. Oculodermal melanocytosis may affect the sclera, and affected patients are at increased risk for glaucoma and ocular melanoma. The presence of scleritis may also be associated with high IOP.

Cornea

Enlargement of the cornea associated with breaks in the Descemet membrane (Haab striae) is commonly found in developmental glaucoma patients. Glaucomas associated with other anterior segment anomalies are described in the following discussions. Punctate epithelial defects, especially in the inferonasal interpalpebral region, are often indicative of medication toxicity. Microcystic epithelial edema is commonly associated with elevated IOP, particularly when the IOP rise is acute. The following corneal endothelial abnormalities can be important clues to underlying associated secondary glaucoma:

- Krukenberg spindle in pigmentary glaucoma
- deposition of exfoliative material in pseudoexfoliation syndrome
- keratic precipitates in uveitic glaucoma
- irregular and vesicular lesions in posterior polymorphous dystrophy
- a "beaten bronze" appearance in the iridocorneal endothelial syndrome
- large posterior embryotoxon in Axenfeld-Rieger syndrome

The clinician should note the presence of traumatic or surgical corneal scars. The central corneal thickness (CCT) of all patients suspected of having glaucoma should be assessed by corneal pachymetry, as a thin central cornea is a risk factor for glaucoma. (See Chapters 2 and 4.)

Anterior chamber

When evaluating the anterior chamber, the examiner should note the uniformity of depth of the chamber and estimate the width of the angle. In the Van Herick method of estimating angle width, the examiner projects a narrow slit beam onto the cornea, just anterior to the limbus. This method may miss narrow angles or angle closure and is not a substitute for gonioscopy, which is discussed in detail later in this chapter.

Iris bombé and plateau iris syndrome can both result in an anterior chamber that is deep centrally and shallow or flat peripherally. In contrast, in malignant (aqueous misdirection) glaucoma and other posterior "pushing" glaucoma mechanisms (see Chapter 1, Fig 1-1), both peripheral and central chambers are shallow. Iris masses, choroidal effusions, or trauma can produce an irregular iris surface contour and nonuniformity or asymmetry in anterior chamber depth. In many circumstances, especially in the assessment of narrow-angle glaucoma, comparing the chamber depth of the 2 eyes is of substantial value. The presence of inflammatory cells, red blood cells, floating pigment, or inflammatory debris (such as fibrin) should be noted. The degree of inflammation (flare and cell) and presence of pigment should be determined before instillation of eyedrops.

Iris

Examination of the iris should be performed before pupillary dilation. The clinician should note heterochromia, iris atrophy, transillumination defects, ectropion uveae, corectopia, nevi, nodules, and exfoliative material. Early stages of neovascularization of the anterior segment may appear as either fine tufts around the pupillary margin or a fine network of vessels on the surface of the iris adjacent to the iris root. The clinician should also examine the iris for evidence of trauma, such as sphincter tears or iridodonesis. Iris color should be noted, especially in patients being considered for treatment with a prostaglandin analogue.

Lens

The clinician should examine the lens both before and after pupillary dilation, evaluating the size, shape, clarity, and stability of the lens. Findings from this examination may help diagnose lens-related glaucomas and guide management. Before the pupil is dilated, phacodonesis, pseudoexfoliation, subluxation, and dislocation should be noted. A posterior subcapsular cataract may be indicative of long-term corticosteroid use. An intraocular foreign body with siderosis and glaucoma may also result in characteristic lens changes. If an intraocular lens is present, the clinician should record its type and position, along with the status of the posterior capsule.

Fundus

A dilated examination allows the clinician to evaluate the vitreous for signs of inflammation, hemorrhage, or ghost cells. Careful stereoscopic evaluation of the optic nerve head should be performed, followed by examination of the fundus to detect posterior segment pathology such as hemorrhages, effusions, masses, inflammatory lesions, retinovascular occlusions, diabetic retinopathy, or retinal detachments that can be associated with the glaucomas.

Gonioscopy

Gonioscopy is an essential diagnostic tool and examination technique used to visualize the structures of the anterior chamber angle (Table 3-1). Unfortunately, this procedure is often underutilized in clinical practice, potentially leading to incorrect diagnosis and

Table 3-1 **Gonioscopic Examination**

Tissue	Features and Pathologic Findings
Posterior cornea	Pigmentation, guttae, corneal endothelium
Schwalbe line	Thickening, anterior displacement
Trabecular meshwork	Pigmentation, peripheral anterior synechiae (PAS), inflammatory or neovascular membranes, keratic precipitates
Scleral spur	Iris processes, presence or absence
Ciliary body band	Width, regularity, cyclodialysis cleft
Iris	Contour, rubeosis, atrophy, cysts, iridodonesis
Pupil and lens	Pseudoexfoliation syndrome, posterior synechiae, position and regularity, sphincter rupture, ectropion uveae
Zonular fibers	Pigmentation, rupture

management. Figures 3-1 and 3-2 give schematic and clinical views of the angle as seen with gonioscopy. Gonioscopy is required in order to visualize the angle because, under normal conditions, light reflected from the angle structures undergoes total internal reflection at the tear–air interface. At the tear–air interface, the critical angle (approximately 46°) is reached, and light is totally reflected back into the corneal stroma. This prevents direct visualization of the angle structures. Gonioscopy lenses eliminate the tear–air interface by placing a plastic or glass surface adjacent to the front surface of the eye. The small space between the lens and cornea is filled by the patient's tears, saline solution, or a clear viscous substance. Depending on the type of lens employed, the angle can be examined with a direct (eg, Koeppe) system or a mirrored indirect (eg, Goldmann or Zeiss) system (Fig 3-3).

Direct and Indirect Gonioscopy

Gonioscopy techniques fall into 1 of 2 broad categories: direct and indirect (see Fig 3-3). *Direct gonioscopy* is performed with a binocular microscope, a fiber-optic illuminator or slit-pen light, and a direct goniolens, such as the Koeppe, Barkan, Wurst, Swan-Jacob, or Richardson lens. The lens is placed on the eye, and saline solution is used to fill the space between the cornea and the lens. The saline acts as an optical coupler between the 2 surfaces. The lens provides direct visualization of the anterior chamber angle (ie, light reflected directly from the angle is visualized). With direct gonioscopy lenses, the clinician has an erect view of the angle structures, which is essential when goniotomies are performed. Direct gonioscopy is most easily performed with the patient in a supine position, and it is commonly used in the operating room for examining the eyes of infants under anesthesia.

Indirect gonioscopy is more frequently used in the clinician's office. Indirect gonioscopy also eliminates the total internal reflection at the surface of the cornea. Light reflected from the angle passes into the indirect gonioscopy lens and is reflected by a mirror within the lens. Indirect gonioscopy may be used with the patient in an upright position, with illumination and magnification provided by a slit lamp. A *goniolens,* which contains 1 or more mirrors, yields an inverted and slightly foreshortened image of the opposite angle. Although the image is inverted with an indirect goniolens, the right–left orientation of a horizontal mirror and the up–down orientation of a vertical mirror remain unchanged. The foreshortening, combined with the upright position of the patient, makes the angle appear a

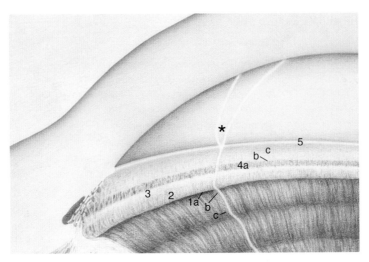

Figure 3-1 Gonioscopic appearance of a normal anterior chamber angle. *1,* Peripheral iris: *a,* insertion; *b,* curvature; *c,* angular approach. *2,* Ciliary body band. *3,* Scleral spur. *4,* Trabecular meshwork: *a,* posterior; *b,* mid; *c,* anterior. *5,* Schwalbe line. *Asterisk,* Corneal optical wedge.

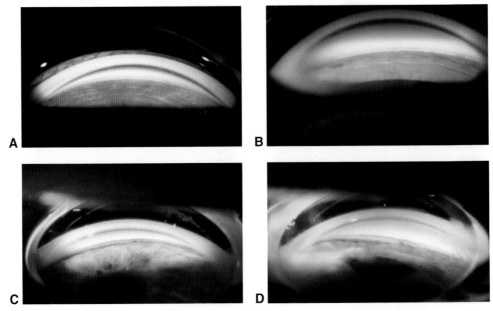

Figure 3-2 Normal and narrow angles. **A,** Normal open angle. Gonioscopic photograph shows trace pigmentation of the posterior trabecular meshwork and normal insertion of the iris into a narrow ciliary body band. The Goldmann lens was used. **B,** Normal open angle. This gonioscopic view using the Goldmann lens shows mild pigmentation of the posterior trabecular meshwork. A wide ciliary body band with posterior insertion of the iris can also be seen. **C,** Narrow angle. This gonioscopic view using the Zeiss lens without indentation shows pigment in the inferior angle but poor visualization of angle anatomy. **D,** Narrow angle. Gonioscopy with a Zeiss lens with indentation shows peripheral anterior synechiae (PAS) in the posterior trabecular meshwork. Pigment deposits on the Schwalbe line can also be seen. This is the same angle as shown in part **C.** *(Courtesy of Elizabeth A. Hodapp, MD.)*

Direct gonioscopy

Indirect

Dynamic

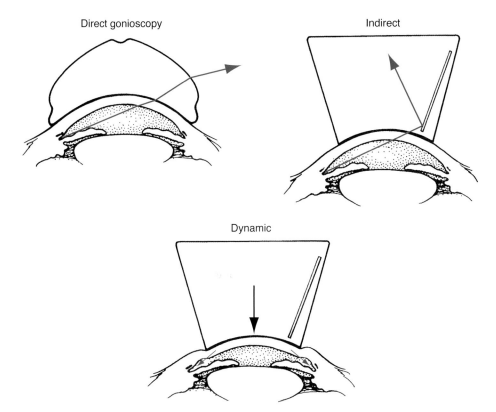

Figure 3-3 Direct and indirect gonioscopy. Gonioscopic lenses eliminate the tear–air interface and total internal reflection. With a direct lens, the light ray reflected from the anterior chamber angle is observed directly, whereas with an indirect lens the light ray is reflected by a mirror within the lens. Posterior pressure with an indirect lens forces open an appositionally closed or narrow anterior chamber angle (dynamic gonioscopy). *(Modified with permission from Wright KW, ed.* Textbook of Ophthalmology. *Baltimore: Williams & Wilkins; 1997.)*

little shallower than it does with direct gonioscopy systems. The Goldmann-type goniolens requires a viscous fluid such as methylcellulose for optical coupling with the cornea. When the goniolens has only 1 mirror, the lens must be rotated to view the entire angle. Posterior pressure on the lens, especially if it is tilted, indents the sclera and may falsely narrow the angle. These lenses provide the clearest visualization of the anterior chamber angle structures, and they may be modified with antireflective coatings for use during laser procedures.

The Posner, Sussman, and Zeiss 4-mirror goniolenses allow all 4 quadrants of the anterior chamber angle to be visualized without rotation of the lens during examination. Since the Goldmann-type lens has approximately the same radius of curvature as the cornea, they are optically coupled by the patient's tears. However, pressure on the cornea may distort the angle. The examiner can detect this pressure by noting the induced Descemet membrane folds. Although pressure may falsely open the angle, the technique of dynamic gonioscopy is sometimes essential for distinguishing iridocorneal apposition from synechial closure. Many clinicians prefer these lenses because of their ease of use and employment in performing dynamic gonioscopy.

Because the posterior diameter of these goniolenses is smaller than the corneal diameter, posterior pressure can be used to force open a narrowed angle. With dynamic gonioscopy (compression or indentation gonioscopy), gentle pressure is placed on the cornea, and aqueous humor is forced into the angle (see Fig 3-3). In inexperienced hands, dynamic gonioscopy may be misleading, as undue pressure on the anterior surface of the cornea may distort the angle or may give the observer the false impression of an open angle. With all indirect gonioscopy techniques, the observer may manipulate the anterior chamber angle by repositioning the patient's eye (having the patient look toward the mirror) or by applying pressure with the posterior surface of the lens to provide more complete evaluation of the angle. However, caution must be used to avoid inducing artificial opening or closing of the angle with these techniques.

Gonioscopic Assessment and Documentation

In performing both direct and indirect gonioscopy, the clinician must recognize the landmarks of the anterior chamber angle. It is important to perform gonioscopy with dim room light and a thin, short light beam in order to minimize the amount of light entering the pupil. An excessive amount of light could result in increased pupillary constriction and a change in the peripheral angle appearance that could falsely open the angle, thereby preventing the correct identification of a narrow or occluded angle. The scleral spur and the Schwalbe line, 2 important angle landmarks, are most consistently identified. A convenient gonioscopic technique to determine the exact position of the Schwalbe line is the *parallelepiped technique*. The parallelepiped, or corneal light wedge, technique allows the observer to determine the exact junction of the cornea and the trabecular meshwork. Using a narrow slit beam and sharp focus, the examiner sees 2 linear reflections, one from the external surface of the cornea and its junction with the sclera and the other from the internal surface of the cornea. The 2 reflections meet at the Schwalbe line (see Fig 3-1). The scleral spur is a thin, pale stripe between the ciliary face and the pigmented zone of the trabecular meshwork. The inferior portion of the angle is generally wider and is the easiest place in which to locate the landmarks. After verifying the landmarks, the clinician should examine the entire angle in an orderly manner (see Table 3-1).

Proper management of glaucoma requires that the clinician determine not only whether the angle is open or closed, but also whether other pathologic findings, such as angle recession or peripheral anterior synechiae (PAS), are present. In angle closure, the peripheral iris obstructs the trabecular meshwork—that is, the meshwork is not visible on gonioscopy. The width of the angle is determined by the site of insertion of the iris on the ciliary face, the convexity of the iris, and the prominence of the peripheral iris roll. In many cases, the angle appears to be open but very narrow. It is often difficult to distinguish a narrow but open angle from an angle with partial closure; dynamic gonioscopy is useful in this situation (see Figs 3-2 and 3-3).

The best method for describing the angle is to use a standardized grading system or draw the iris contour, the location of the iris insertion, and the angle between the iris and the trabecular meshwork. A variety of gonioscopic grading systems have been developed, all of which facilitate standardized description of angle structures and abbreviate that description. Keep in mind that, with abbreviated descriptions, some details of the angle structure will be eliminated. The most commonly used gonioscopic grading systems are the Shaffer and Spaeth systems. A quadrant-by-quadrant narrative description of the chamber angle noting localized findings such as neovascular tufts, angle recession, or PAS may also be used to document serial gonioscopic findings. If a grading system is used, the clinician should specify which system is being used.

The *Shaffer system* describes the angle between the trabecular meshwork and the iris as follows:

- *Grade 4:* The angle between the iris and the surface of the trabecular meshwork is 45°.
- *Grade 3:* The angle between the iris and the surface of the trabecular meshwork is greater than 20° but less than 45°.
- *Grade 2:* The angle between the iris and the surface of the trabecular meshwork is 20°. Angle closure is possible.
- *Grade 1:* The angle between the iris and the surface of the trabecular meshwork is 10°. Angle closure is probable in time.
- *Slit:* The angle between the iris and the surface of the trabecular meshwork is less than 10°. Angle closure is very likely.
- *0:* The iris is against the trabecular meshwork. Angle closure is present.

The *Spaeth gonioscopic grading system* expands this system to include a description of the peripheral iris contour, the insertion of the iris root, and the effects of dynamic gonioscopy on the angle configuration (Fig 3-4).

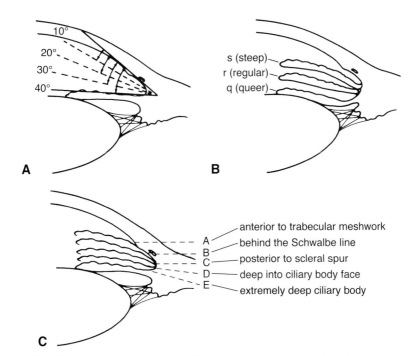

Figure 3-4 The Spaeth gonioscopic classification of the anterior chamber angle, based on 3 variables: angular width of the angle recess **(A)**; configuration of the peripheral iris **(B)**; and apparent insertion of the iris root **(C)**. *(Reproduced with permission from Shields MB.* Textbook of Glaucoma. *3rd ed. Baltimore: Williams & Wilkins; 1992.)*

Ordinarily, the Schlemm canal is invisible by gonioscopy. However, blood enters the Schlemm canal when episcleral venous pressure exceeds IOP, most commonly because of compression of the episcleral veins by the lip of the goniolens (Fig 3-5). Pathologic causes include hypotony and elevated episcleral venous pressure, as in carotid-cavernous fistula or Sturge-Weber syndrome.

Normal blood vessels in the angle include radial iris vessels, portions of the arterial circle of the ciliary body, and vertical branches of the anterior ciliary arteries. Normal vessels are oriented either radially along the iris or circumferentially (in a serpentine manner) in the ciliary body face. Vessels that cross the scleral spur to reach the trabecular meshwork are usually abnormal (Fig 3-6). The vessels seen in Fuchs heterochromic uveitis are fine, branching, unsheathed, and meandering. Patients with neovascular glaucoma have

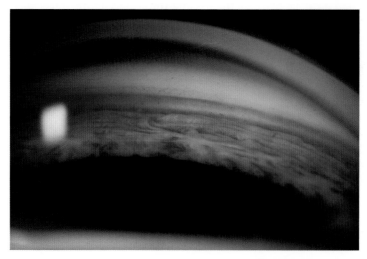

Figure 3-5 Goniophotograph showing blood in Schlemm canal. Note the red line posterior to the trabecular meshwork in this patient with elevated episcleral venous pressure resulting in blood reflux into the Schlemm canal. *(Courtesy of G. A. Cioffi, MD.)*

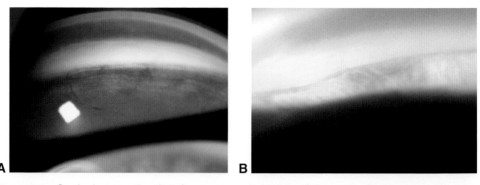

A   B

Figure 3-6 Goniophotographs showing neovascularization of the angle. **A,** Anatomically open angle. **B,** Closed angle. *(Part A courtesy of Keith Barton, MD; part B courtesy of Ronald L. Gross, MD.)*

trunklike vessels crossing the ciliary body and scleral spur and arborizing over the trabecular meshwork. Contraction of the myofibroblasts accompanying these vessels leads to PAS formation.

It is important to distinguish PAS from iris processes (the uveal meshwork), which are open and lacy and follow the normal curve of the angle. The angle structures are visible in the open spaces between the processes. Synechiae are more solid or sheetlike (Fig 3-7). They are composed of iris stroma and obliterate the angle recess.

Pigmentation of the trabecular meshwork increases with age and tends to be more marked in individuals with darkly pigmented irides. Pigmentation can be segmental and is usually most marked in the inferior angle. The pigmentation pattern of an individual angle is dynamic over time, especially in conditions such as pigment dispersion syndrome. Heavy pigmentation of the trabecular meshwork should suggest pigment dispersion or pseudoexfoliation syndrome. Pseudoexfoliation syndrome may appear clinically similar to pigment dispersion syndrome, with pigment granules on the anterior surface of the iris, increased pigment in the anterior chamber angle, and secondary open-angle glaucoma. In addition, a line of pigment deposition anterior to the Schwalbe line is often present in pseudoexfoliation syndrome (Sampaolesi line). Other conditions that cause increased anterior chamber angle pigmentation include melanoma, trauma, surgery, inflammation, angle closure, and hyphema.

Posttraumatic angle recession may be associated with monocular open-angle glaucoma. The gonioscopic criteria for diagnosing angle recession include

- an abnormally wide ciliary body band (Fig 3-8)
- increased prominence of the scleral spur
- torn iris processes
- marked variation of ciliary face width and angle depth in different quadrants of the same eye

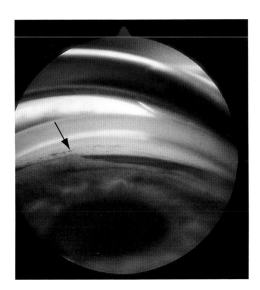

Figure 3-7 Goniophotograph showing both an area of sheetlike PAS *(arrow)* and an open angle *(right)*. *(Courtesy of Louis B. Cantor, MD.)*

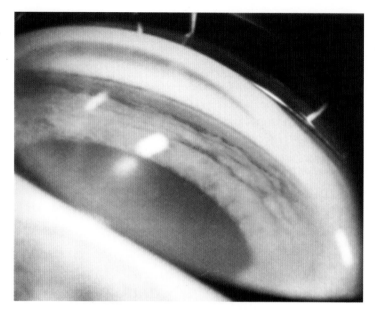

Figure 3-8 Goniophotograph showing angle recession. Note the widening of the ciliary body band. *(Reprinted with permission from Wright KW, ed.* Textbook of Ophthalmology. *Baltimore: Williams & Wilkins; 1997.)*

In evaluating for angle recession, the clinician may find it helpful to compare one part of the angle to other areas in the same eye or to the same area in the fellow eye.

Figure 3-9 illustrates the variety of gonioscopic findings caused by blunt trauma. If the ciliary body separates from the scleral spur (cyclodialysis), it will appear gonioscopically as a deep angle recess with a gap between the scleral spur and the ciliary body. Detection of a very small cleft may require ultrasound biomicroscopy.

Other findings that may be visible by gonioscopy are

- microhyphema or hypopyon
- retained anterior chamber foreign body
- iridodialysis
- sclerostomy site and tube shunts
- angle precipitates suggestive of glaucomatocyclitic crisis
- pigmentation of the lens equator
- other peripheral lens abnormalities
- intraocular lens haptics
- ciliary body tumors/cyst

Alward WLM. *Color Atlas of Gonioscopy.* 2nd ed. San Francisco: Foundation of the American Academy of Ophthalmology; 2008.

Savage JA. Gonioscopy in the management of glaucoma. *Focal Points: Clinical Modules for Ophthalmologists.* San Francisco: American Academy of Ophthalmology; 2006, module 3.

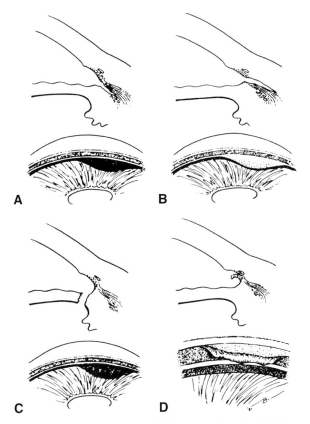

Figure 3-9 Forms of anterior chamber angle injury associated with blunt trauma, showing cross-sectional and corresponding gonioscopic appearance. **A,** Angle recession (tear between longitudinal and circular muscles of ciliary body). **B,** Cyclodialysis (separation of ciliary body from scleral spur) with widening of suprachoroidal space. **C,** Iridodialysis (tear in root of iris). **D,** Trabecular damage (tear in anterior portion of meshwork, creating a flap that is hinged at the scleral spur). *(Reproduced with permission from Shields MB.* Textbook of Glaucoma. *3rd ed. Baltimore: Williams & Wilkins; 1992.)*

The Optic Nerve

The entire visual pathway is described and illustrated in BCSC Section 5, *Neuro-Ophthalmology.* For further discussion of retinal involvement in the visual process, see Section 12, *Retina and Vitreous.*

Anatomy and Pathology

The optic nerve is the neural connection between the neurosensory retina and the brain, primarily the lateral geniculate body. An understanding of the normal and pathologic appearance of the optic nerve allows the clinician to detect glaucoma, as well as to follow glaucoma cases. The optic nerve is composed of neural tissue, glial tissue, extracellular matrix, and blood vessels. The human optic nerve consists of approximately 1.2–1.5 million axons of retinal ganglion cells (RGCs), although there is significant individual variability. The cell bodies of the RGCs lie in the ganglion cell layer of the retina. The intraorbital optic nerve is divided into 2 components: the anterior optic nerve and the posterior optic nerve. The anterior optic nerve extends from the retinal surface to the retrolaminar region, just where the nerve exits the posterior aspect of the globe. The average diameter of the optic nerve head is approximately 1.5–1.7 mm as measured with planimetry, but it varies widely among individuals and ethnic groups; the optic nerve expands to approximately 3–4 mm immediately upon exiting the globe. The increase in size is accounted for by axonal myelination, glial tissue, and the beginning of the leptomeninges (optic nerve sheath). The axons are separated into fascicles within the optic nerve, with the intervening spaces occupied by astrocytes.

In primates, there are 3 major RGC types involved in conscious visual perception: magnocellular neurons (M cells), parvocellular neurons (P cells), and koniocellular neurons (bistratified cells). M cells have large-diameter axons, synapse in the magnocellular layer of the lateral geniculate body, are sensitive to luminance changes in dim illumination (scotopic conditions), have the largest dendritic field, primarily process information related to motion perception, and are not responsive to color. In comparison to the M cells, the P cells account for approximately 80% of all ganglion cells; they are concentrated in the central retina; and they have smaller-diameter axons, smaller receptive fields, and slower conduction velocity. They synapse in the parvocellular layers of the lateral geniculate body. P cells subserve color vision, are most active under higher luminance conditions, and discriminate fine detail. The cells are motion-insensitive and process information of high spatial frequency (high resolution). The bistratified cells (koniocellular neurons) process information concerned with blue-yellow color opponency. This system, which is likely preferentially activated by short-wavelength perimetry, is inhibited when red and green cones (yellow) are activated and stimulated when blue cones are activated. Bistratified and large M cells each account for approximately 10% of RGCs.

The distribution of nerve fibers as they enter the optic nerve head is shown in Figure 3-10. The arcuate nerve fibers entering the superior and inferior poles of the disc seem to be more susceptible to glaucomatous damage. This susceptibility explains the frequent occurrence of arcuate nerve fiber bundle visual field defects in glaucoma. The arrangement of the axons in the optic nerve head and their differential susceptibility to damage determine the patterns of visual field loss seen in glaucoma, which are described and illustrated later in this chapter.

The anterior optic nerve can be divided into 4 layers:

- nerve fiber
- prelaminar
- laminar
- retrolaminar

The most anterior zone is the superficial nerve fiber layer region, which is continuous with the *nerve fiber layer* of the retina. This region is primarily composed of the axons of the RGCs in transition from the superficial retina to the neuronal component of the optic

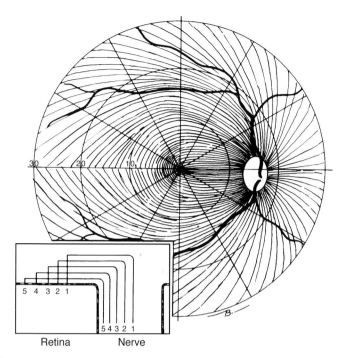

Figure 3-10 Anatomy of retinal nerve fiber distribution. Inset depicts cross-sectional view of axonal arrangement. Peripheral fibers run closer to the choroid and exit in the periphery of the optic nerve, while fibers originating closer to the nerve head are situated closer to the vitreous and occupy a more central portion of the nerve. *(Reproduced with permission from Shields MB.* Textbook of Glaucoma. *3rd ed. Baltimore: Williams & Wilkins; 1992.)*

nerve. The nerve fiber layer can be viewed with the ophthalmoscope when the red-free (green) filter is used. Immediately posterior to the nerve fiber layer is the *prelaminar region,* which lies adjacent to the peripapillary choroid. More posteriorly, the *laminar region* is continuous with the sclera and is composed of the lamina cribrosa, a structure consisting of fenestrated connective tissue lamellae that allow the transit of neural fibers through the scleral coat. Finally, the *retrolaminar region* lies posterior to the lamina cribrosa, is marked by the beginning of axonal myelination, and is surrounded by the leptomeninges of the central nervous system.

The lamina cribrosa provides the main structural support for the optic nerve as it exits the eye and is composed of a reticulated network of connective tissue beams that are composed primarily of collagen (Fig 3-11). Other extracellular matrix components include elastin, laminin, and fibronectin. Beams also contain the capillaries that nourish this critical region. Neural components of the optic nerve pass through these connective tissue beams. In addition, relatively large, central fenestrations allow transit of the central retinal artery and central retinal vein. The connective tissue density within the lamina has been described histologically as lesser superiorly and inferiorly as compared with the temporal and nasal aspects of the optic nerve. It has been suggested that these differences play a role in the development of glaucomatous optic neuropathy. The pores of the lamina cribrosa may often be seen by ophthalmoscopy at the base of the optic nerve head cup.

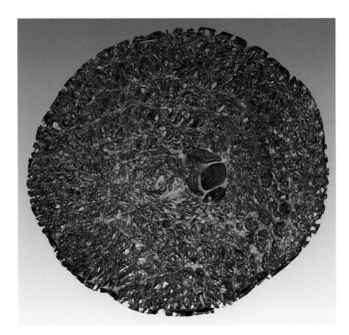

Figure 3-11 Anterior view of the human lamina cribrosa from a healthy donor, obtained from 3-dimensional episcopic autofluorescent reconstruction illustrating the reticular network of supportive connective tissue. *(Courtesy of Crawford Downs, PhD, and Christopher Girkin, MD.)*

Between the optic nerve and the adjacent choroidal and scleral tissue lies a rim of connective tissue, the ring of Elschnig.

> Downs JC. Optic nerve head biomechanics in aging and disease. *Exp Eye Res.* 2015;133: 19–29.

Blood supply to the optic nerve

The vascular anatomy of the anterior optic nerve and peripapillary region has been extensively studied (Fig 3-12). The arterial supply of the anterior optic nerve is derived entirely from branches of the ophthalmic artery via 1–5 posterior ciliary arteries. Typically, between 2 and 4 posterior ciliary arteries course anteriorly before dividing into approximately 10–20 short posterior ciliary arteries prior to entering the posterior globe. Often, the posterior ciliary arteries separate into a medial and a lateral group before branching into the short posterior ciliary arteries. The short posterior ciliary arteries penetrate the perineural sclera of the posterior globe to supply the peripapillary choroid, as well as most of the anterior optic nerve. Some short posterior ciliary arteries course, without branching, through the sclera directly into the choroid; others divide within the sclera to provide branches to both the choroid and the optic nerve. Often a noncontinuous arterial circle exists within the perineural sclera, the circle of Zinn-Haller. The central retinal artery, also a posterior orbital branch of the ophthalmic artery, penetrates the optic nerve approximately 10–15 mm behind the globe. The central retinal artery has few, if any, intraneural branches, the exception being an occasional small branch within the retrolaminar region, which may anastomose with the pial system. The central retinal artery courses adjacent to the central retinal vein within the central portion of the optic nerve.

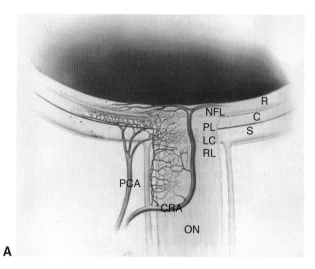

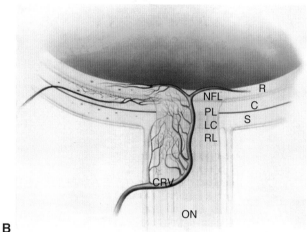

Figure 3-12 Anterior optic nerve vasculature. **A,** Arterial supply to the anterior optic nerve and peripapillary choroid. Lamina cribrosa (LC), superficial nerve fiber layer (NFL), prelamina (PL), retrolamina (RL), central retinal artery (CRA), optic nerve (ON), choroid (C), posterior ciliary artery (PCA), retina (R), sclera (S). **B,** Venous drainage of the anterior optic nerve and peripapillary choroid. Lamina cribrosa (LC), nerve fiber layer (NFL), prelamina (PL), retrolamina (RL), choroid (C), retina (R), sclera (S), optic nerve (ON), central retinal vein (CRV). *(Reprinted with permission from Wright KW, ed.* Textbook of Ophthalmology. *Baltimore: Williams & Wilkins; 1997:592, Figs 44-2, 44-3.)*

The superficial nerve fiber layer is supplied principally by recurrent retinal arterioles branching from the central retinal artery. These small vessels, originating in the peripapillary nerve fiber layer, run toward the center of the optic nerve head and have been referred to as *epipapillary vessels.* The capillary branches from these vessels are continuous with the retinal capillaries at the optic nerve head margin, but they also have posterior anastomoses with the prelaminar capillaries of the optic nerve. The temporal nerve fiber layer may have an arterial contribution from the cilioretinal artery, when it is present.

The *prelaminar region* is principally supplied by direct branches of the short posterior ciliary arteries and by branches of the circle of Zinn-Haller, when it is present. In eyes with a well-developed circle of Zinn-Haller, arterial branches emerge to supply both the prelaminar and the laminar regions. The lamina cribrosa region also receives its blood supply from branches of the short posterior ciliary arteries or from branches of the circle of Zinn-Haller; this is similar to the prelaminar region. These precapillary branches perforate the outer aspects of the lamina cribrosa before branching into an intraseptal capillary network. Arterioles also branch from the short posterior ciliary arteries and the circle of Zinn-Haller and course posteriorly to supply the pial arteries. These pial arteries often contribute to the laminar region. As in the prelaminar region, the larger vessels of the peripapillary choroid may contribute occasional small arterioles to this region, although there is no connection between the peripapillary choriocapillaris and the capillaries of the optic nerve.

The *retrolaminar region* is also supplied by branches from the short posterior ciliary arteries, as well as by the pial arterial branches coursing adjacent to the retrolaminar optic nerve region. The pial arteries originate from both the central retinal artery, before it pierces the retrobulbar optic nerve, and branches of the short posterior ciliary arteries more anteriorly. The central retinal artery may supply several small intraneural branches in the retrolaminar region.

The rich capillary beds of each of the 4 anatomical regions within the anterior optic nerve are anatomically confluent. The venous drainage of the anterior optic nerve is almost exclusively via a single vein, the central retinal vein. In the nerve fiber layer, blood is drained directly into the retinal veins, which then join to form the central retinal vein. In the prelaminar, laminar, and retrolaminar regions, venous drainage also occurs via the central retinal vein or axial tributaries to the central retinal vein.

Mackenzie PJ, Cioffi GA. Vascular anatomy of the optic nerve head. *Can J Ophthalmol.* 2008; 43(3):308–312.

Glaucomatous Optic Neuropathy

Glaucomatous optic neuropathy is the sine qua non of all forms of glaucoma (Fig 3-13). Histologically, early glaucomatous cupping consists of loss of axons, blood vessels, and glial cells. The loss of tissue seems to start at the level of the lamina cribrosa and is associated with remodeling of the load-bearing connective tissues. It is most pronounced at the superior and inferior poles of the optic nerve head. In many cases, though not always, structural optic nerve changes may precede detectable functional loss.

Glaucomatous cupping in infants and children is accompanied by an expansion of the entire scleral ring, which may explain why cupping seems to occur earlier in children and why reversibility of cupping is more prominent with successful treatment in these cases. Cupping may be reversed in adults as well, but such reversal is less frequent and more subtle.

Glaucomatous optic neuropathy is a progressive degeneration of RGCs and their axons, with damage extending from the optic nerve to the major visual centers in the brain, such as the lateral geniculate nucleus. IOP plays a major role in the development of glaucomatous optic neuropathy in most individuals and is considered the most significant risk factor. The role of IOP as a risk factor for development and progression in glaucoma

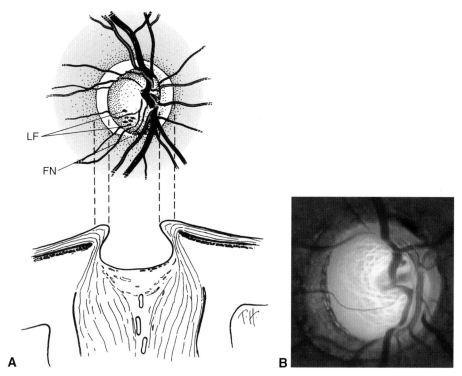

LF

FN

A

B

Figure 3-13 Two views of glaucomatous optic nerves. **A,** Glaucomatous optic nerve (anterior optic nerve head and transverse view, right eye). Note thinning, undermining, and focal notching (FN) of inferior neuroretinal rim; enlarged central cup with visible laminar fenestrations (LF); nasal shift of retinal vessels; and peripapillary atrophy. **B,** Clinical view of glaucomatous optic nerve head demonstrating extensive loss of the neuroretinal rim. *(Part A reprinted with permission from Wright KW, ed.* Textbook of Ophthalmology. *Baltimore: Williams & Wilkins; 1997. Part B courtesy of Ronald L. Gross, MD.)*

has been well established by several multicenter randomized clinical trials, as well as by experimental investigations. However, up to one-third of patients in North America have signs of glaucomatous damage to the optic nerve despite IOP levels within statistically normal limits. Therefore, it is likely that factors other than IOP may contribute to a given individual's susceptibility to glaucomatous damage.

Damage from direct compression of axonal fibers, with distortion of the lamina cribrosa beams and interruption of axoplasmic flow, may contribute to RGC death. Decreased optic nerve head perfusion and/or disturbance of vascular autoregulation may also contribute to optic nerve damage in glaucoma, either directly or as a consequence of biomechanical effects. Alternatively, changes in systemic hemodynamics may result in perfusion deficits, even at a normal IOP level. Neural degeneration in glaucoma may have a number of triggers. Glutamate excitotoxicity, autoimmunity, and neurotrophic deprivation have all been suggested as causes of secondary injury. Current thinking recognizes that glaucoma is a heterogeneous family of disorders mediated, most likely, by many factors.

Weinreb RN, Aung T, Medeiros FA. The pathophysiology and treatment of glaucoma: A review. *JAMA.* 2014;311(18):1901–1911.

Examination of the Optic Nerve Head

Clinical examination of the optic nerve head is preferably performed with a slit-lamp biomicroscope combined with a high-magnification posterior pole lens (60.00, 78.00, or 90.00 D lens). The slit beam, rather than diffuse illumination, is useful for determining subtle changes in the contour of the nerve head. This system provides high magnification, excellent illumination, and a stereoscopic view of the optic nerve head. This also allows for quantitative measurement of the diameter of the optic nerve head, by adjusting the height of the slit beam. The disc is viewed through the handheld lens until the height of the slit is the same as the vertical diameter of the disc. The disc diameter can then be calculated by taking into account the lens used. With a 60.00 D lens, the height of the slit equals the disc diameter, in millimeters, read directly from the scale. If a 78.00 D lens is used, the scale reading is multiplied by 1.1, and with a 90.00 D lens multiplication by 1.3 results in the disc diameter in millimeters. The normal-sized optic nerve head ranges from approximately 1.5 to 2.2 mm in diameter.

The *direct ophthalmoscope* also may be used for clinical examination of the optic nerve head. However, this instrument may not provide sufficient stereoscopic detail to detect subtle changes in optic nerve head topography. The *indirect ophthalmoscope* can be used for examination of the optic nerve head in young children and in uncooperative patients. With the indirect ophthalmoscope, cupping of the optic nerve can be detected, but, in general, optic nerve cupping and pallor appear less pronounced than with slit-lamp methods, and the magnification is often inadequate for detecting subtle or localized details important in the evaluation of glaucoma. Thus, the indirect ophthalmoscope is not recommended for routine use in examining the optic nerve head.

The optic nerve head is usually round or slightly oval in shape and contains a central *cup*. The tissue between the cup and the disc margin is called the *neural rim* or *neuroretinal rim*. In individuals without glaucoma, the rim has a relatively uniform width and a color that ranges from orange to pink. The size of the physiologic cup is developmentally determined and is related to the size of the disc. For a given number of nerve fibers, the larger the overall disc area, the larger the cup. Cup–disc ratio alone is not an adequate assessment of the optic nerve head for possible glaucomatous damage. For example, a 0.7 ratio in a large optic nerve head may be normal, whereas a 0.3 ratio in a very small disc could be pathologic. This shows the importance of assessing the disc size. The size of the cup may increase slightly with age. Nonglaucomatous black individuals, on average, have larger disc areas and larger cup–disc ratios than do whites, although a substantial overlap exists.

Differentiating physiologic or normal cupping from acquired *glaucomatous cupping* of the optic nerve head can be difficult. The early changes of glaucomatous optic neuropathy are very subtle and include generalized enlargement of the cup, focal rim thinning, superficial disc hemorrhage, nerve fiber layer loss, asymmetry of cupping, and beta (β) zone of peripapillary atrophy (Table 3-2).

Diffuse neuroretinal rim thinning associated with generalized enlargement of the cup may be an early sign of glaucomatous damage. However, diffuse loss may be difficult to appreciate unless previous objective documentation of the optic nerve head (eg, photographs) is available. Comparing one eye with the fellow eye may be helpful, because cup asymmetry is unusual in normal eyes in the absence of disc size asymmetry (Fig 3-14).

Table 3-2 Ophthalmoscopic Signs of Glaucoma

Generalized	Focal	Less Specific
Large optic cup Asymmetry of the cups Progressive enlargement of the cup	Notching of the rim Vertical elongation of the cup Cupping to the rim margin Nerve fiber layer hemorrhage Nerve fiber layer loss	Exposed lamina cribrosa Nasal displacement of vessels Baring of circumlinear vessels Peripapillary atrophy

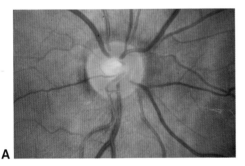 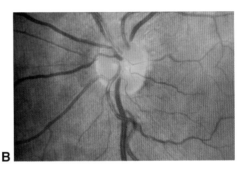

A   B

Figure 3-14 Optic nerve head photograph showing asymmetry of optic nerve cupping. Note the generalized enlargement of the cup in the right eye **(A)** as compared with the left eye **(B)**. Asymmetry of the cup–disc ratio of more than 0.2 occurs in less than 1% of individuals without glaucoma. *(Courtesy of G. A. Cioffi, MD.)*

The vertical cup–disc ratio is normally between 0.1 and 0.4, although as many as 5% of individuals without glaucoma will have cup–disc ratios larger than 0.6. Asymmetry of the cup–disc ratio of more than 0.2 occurs in less than 1% of individuals without glaucoma. This asymmetry may be related to disc size asymmetry. Increased size of the physiologic cup may be a familial trait, and it is also seen with high myopia. An oblique insertion of the optic nerve into the globe of individuals with high myopia may also cause a tilted appearance to the optic nerve head. Examination of other family members may clarify whether a large cup is inherited or acquired.

Localized loss of the neuroretinal rim most typically occurs at the inferior and superior temporal poles of the optic nerve in early glaucomatous optic neuropathy. The preferential loss of rim tissue in the superior and inferior poles leads to a vertically elongated cup in glaucomatous nerves (Fig 3-15). To help identify subtle thinning of the neuroretinal rim, a convention referred to as the *ISNT rule* may be useful. In normal eyes, the *Inferior* neuroretinal rim is generally the thickest, followed by the *Superior* rim, the *Nasal* rim, and finally the *Temporal* rim. Therefore, if the rim widths do not follow this pattern, there should be increased concern for the presence of focal loss of rim tissue. However, violation of the ISNT rule is not highly specific and may be seen in normal eyes as well. Deep localized notching, where the lamina cribrosa is visible at the disc margin, is sometimes termed an *acquired optic disc pit*. Patients with acquired pits are at especially high risk for progression. Even in the normal eye, laminar trabeculations or pores may be seen as grayish dots in the base of the physiologic cup. With glaucomatous optic neuropathy, neural atrophy

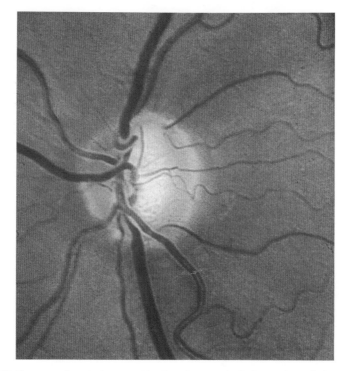

Figure 3-15 Optic nerve head photograph showing vertical elongation of the cup with localized thinning of the inferior and superior neuroretinal rim in the left eye of a patient with moderately advanced glaucoma. *(Courtesy of Felipe A. Medeiros, MD, PhD.)*

results in more extensive exposure of the underlying lamina cribrosa and may reveal more laminar pores or striations in the optic nerve cup. Nasalization of the central retinal artery and central retinal vein is often seen as the cup enlarges.

Although *nerve fiber layer hemorrhages* usually appear as a linear red streak on or near the disc surface (Fig 3-16), their appearance is highly variable. One-third of glaucoma patients at some time during the course of their disease may develop hemorrhages, which typically clear over several weeks to months. They are often followed by localized notching of the rim and visual field loss. Some glaucoma patients have repeated episodes of optic disc hemorrhage; others have none. Optic nerve head hemorrhage is an important prognostic sign for the development or progression of visual field loss, and any patient with a disc hemorrhage requires detailed evaluation and follow-up. Disc hemorrhages may also be caused by posterior vitreous detachments, diabetes mellitus, branch retinal vein occlusions, and anticoagulation therapy.

Axons in the nerve fiber layer of the normal eye may best be visualized with red-free illumination. As the nerve fibers extend from the peripheral retina to converge at the optic nerve head, they appear as fine striations created by the bundles of axons. In the healthy eye, the brightness and striations of the nerve fiber layer are more easily visible superiorly and inferiorly. With progressive glaucomatous optic neuropathy, the nerve fiber layer thins and becomes less visible. The loss may be diffuse (generalized) or localized (Fig 3-17).

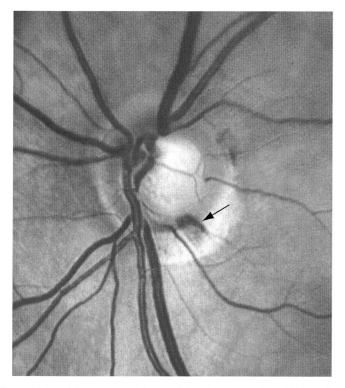

Figure 3-16 Flame-shaped hemorrhage in the left optic nerve head *(arrow)* at the 5-o'clock position in a patient with open-angle glaucoma. *(Courtesy of Felipe A. Medeiros, MD, PhD.)*

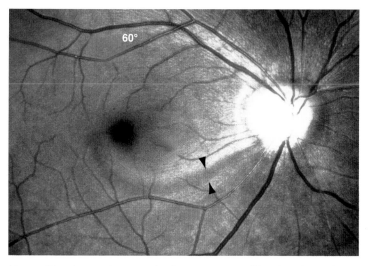

Figure 3-17 Nerve fiber layer photograph shows a nerve fiber bundle defect *(arrowheads)*. *(Courtesy of Louis B. Cantor, MD.)*

With diffuse loss, there is general reduction of the retinal nerve fiber layer (RNFL) brightness, with reduction of the difference normally occurring between the superior and inferior poles, when compared to the temporal and nasal regions. Localized RNFL loss appears as wedge-shaped dark areas emanating from the optic nerve head in an arcuate pattern. Slitlike defects can sometimes also be seen in the nerve fiber layer; however, these are seen in normal RNFL anatomy, though usually not extending to the disc margin. Early wedge-shaped defects are sometimes visible only at a distance from the optic disc margin. *Diffuse nerve fiber loss* is more common in glaucoma than is focal loss but also more difficult to observe. The nerve fiber layer can be visualized clearly in high-contrast black-and-white photographs, and experienced observers can recognize even early disease if good-quality photographs are available. Slit-lamp techniques and direct ophthalmoscopy can be successfully employed to observe the RNFL. The combination of red-free filter, wide slit beam, and posterior pole lens at the slit lamp affords the best view.

There are 2 types of peripapillary atrophy (PPA): alpha (α) zone and beta (β) zone. Alpha zone is present in most normal eyes as well as in eyes with glaucoma and is characterized by a region of irregular hypopigmentation and hyperpigmentation of the retinal pigment epithelium (RPE). The more important zone with respect to glaucoma is β zone, which is due to atrophy of the RPE and choriocapillaris, leading to increased visibility of the large choroidal vessels and sclera. Beta zone is more common and extensive in eyes with glaucoma than in healthy eyes. The area of PPA is spatially correlated with the area of neuroretinal rim loss, with the atrophy being largest in the corresponding area of thinner neuroretinal rim. Therefore, an area of β-zone atrophy should draw the examiner's attention to the adjacent neuroretinal rim to search for glaucomatous loss.

Other, less specific, signs of glaucomatous damage include nasal displacement of the vessels, narrowing of peripapillary retinal vessels, and baring of the circumlinear vessels. With advanced damage, the cup becomes pale and markedly excavated.

It is important to recognize that glaucomatous optic nerve damage is only one type of pathologic change of the optic nerve; other etiologies of optic nerve changes should be considered in the differential diagnosis. Certain conditions may cause apparent cupping of the optic nerve that can be confounded with glaucoma, such as congenital pits of the optic nerve head, coloboma, morning glory syndrome, arteritic ischemic neuropathy or compressive optic neuropathies. Optic nerve heads in which the remaining neuroretinal rim tissue is pale may need to be evaluated for causes of nonglaucomatous optic atrophy (see BCSC Section 5, *Neuro-Ophthalmology*). With rare exceptions, glaucoma results in increased cupping and pallor within the cup, but not pallor of the remaining rim tissue. However, rim pallor out of proportion to the degree of cupping may sometimes occur following previous episodes of very high IOP elevation, such as following an episode of acute angle closure. The ophthalmologist must also consider drusen or coloboma as possible causes of optic nerve change and visual field loss. Finally, the myopic optic disc represents a challenge when the ophthalmologist is attempting to assess possible glaucomatous damage. The size, tilting, and associated structural changes often preclude the ability to definitively determine the presence of glaucomatous damage.

Jonas JB, Budde WM, Panda-Jonas S. Ophthalmoscopic evaluation of the optic nerve head. *Surv Ophthalmol.* 1999;43(4):293–320.

Recording of optic nerve findings

Due to the large variability in the appearance of the optic nerve head in healthy subjects, it is frequently not possible to confirm the presence of glaucomatous damage based on a single cross-sectional observation. Therefore, glaucoma diagnosis frequently requires longitudinal monitoring and detection of progressive damage over time. Careful documentation is essential in order to allow adequate comparison of the optic nerve head appearance over time, both for diagnosis of the disease in individuals suspected of having glaucoma, and for detection of progression in those with established disease.

It is common practice to grade an optic nerve head by comparing the diameter of the cup with the diameter of the disc. This ratio is usually expressed as a decimal, for example, 0.2; but such a description poorly conveys the appearance of the nerve head. A detailed, annotated diagram of the optic nerve head topography is preferable to the recording of a simple cup–disc ratio. The diagram must be of adequate size to allow depiction of important topographic landmarks and morphologic features. With annotation, the diagram can convey the cup–disc ratio along all dimensions and serves to document the presence or absence of regions of rim thinning, notching, hemorrhage, and peripapillary atrophy. However, even very well-detailed descriptions or drawings of the optic nerve head are generally insufficient to detect the subtle changes that may occur as the result of glaucomatous progression over time. Therefore, objective documentation of the appearance of the optic nerve head by photographs or imaging should be obtained whenever possible.

Photography, particularly simultaneous stereophotography, is an excellent method for recording the appearance of the optic nerve for detailed examination and sequential follow-up. This record allows the examiner to compare the present status of the patient with the baseline status without resorting to memory or grading systems. If stereoscopic photographs are not available, even simple monoscopic photographs are preferable to drawings in documenting the appearance of the optic nerve head. However, evaluation of optic nerve head photographs is subjective and does not provide direct quantitative information about the degree of neural loss or rates of disease progression.

Imaging of the optic nerve head and retinal nerve fiber layer

Since the 1850s, the appearance of the optic nerve head has been recognized as critical in assessing the disease status of glaucoma. However, assessment of the optic nerve head at the slit-lamp or through photographs is subjective and shows relatively large interobserver and intraobserver variation. Advancements in ocular imaging technologies over the last 3 decades include optical coherence tomography (OCT), confocal scanning laser ophthalmoscopy (CSLO), and scanning laser polarimetry (SLP). Imaging devices provide an objective means to obtain reproducible and high-resolution images of ocular structures relevant to glaucoma. In addition, imaging devices contain normative databases that allow one to determine the probability that observed measurements are within the normal range, assisting in the differentiation of optic nerve damage from normal variation. Imaging assessment is also helpful for detecting progressive structural damage and for assessment of rates of disease progression.

Of current imaging technologies, OCT offers the greatest versatility and has evolved considerably since first used to image the eye in 1991. OCT employs the principles of low-coherence interferometry and is analogous to ultrasound B-mode imaging, but it uses light instead of sound to acquire high-resolution images of ocular structures. The original OCT technology of time-domain OCT (TD-OCT) has been superseded by Fourier- or spectral-domain OCT (SD-OCT), which has improved spatial resolution and image acquisition speed, resulting in enhanced image quality and greater reproducibility. OCT is able to provide measurements of the peripapillary RNFL thickness, which have been shown to discriminate glaucomatous from healthy eyes. OCT RNFL thickness measurements are in general decreased in glaucomatous eyes compared to those in normal eyes, although considerable inter-individual variability exists. Measurements parameters obtained by OCT have generally included the global average peripapillary RNFL thickness, corresponding to the average of all thickness measurements in a peripapillary circle around the optic nerve head, as well as parameters measuring thickness by quadrants (superior, inferior, temporal, nasal) or in small clock-hour sectors. Figure 3-18 shows an example of RNFL analysis provided by SD-OCT in a patient with glaucomatous RNFL loss in the right eye and normal RNFL in the left eye. RNFL analysis with OCT has also been shown to detect glaucomatous damage in some eyes before the appearance of visual field defects on standard automated perimetry (Fig 3-19) and to be predictive of development of future visual field losses in glaucoma suspect eyes.

In recent years, increased attention has been directed toward the macular region for evaluation of glaucomatous damage. As a large proportion of total macular thickness is composed of RNFL and ganglion cell bodies, this region is an attractive area for identifying structural damage from the disease. The macular RGC layer contains more than 50% of the RGCs of the entire retina. Investigations have also suggested that, in contrary to previous belief, glaucomatous damage frequently affects the macular region, leading to central visual field losses that can go undetected with conventional perimetry.

SD-OCT allows quantitative assessment of either the entire macular thickness or the thickness of specific layers that may be important in glaucoma. Parameters available from SD-OCT analysis of the macular area include, for example, the macular RNFL, the ganglion cell layer with the inner plexiform layer (GCIPL), and the so-called *ganglion cell complex (GCC),* which has been described as comprising the RNFL, the ganglion cell layer, and the inner plexiform layer. Macular parameters are able to distinguish glaucomatous eyes from those of healthy subjects; however, their additional benefit over peripapillary RNFL assessment is still not well established. In eyes with myopic discs or large areas of peripapillary atrophy, which can present with artifacts on peripapillary RNFL assessment, it is likely that macular evaluation may provide increased ability to diagnose and monitor glaucomatous damage. SD-OCT is also able to provide tridimensional topographical measurements of the optic nerve head, including optic nerve head area, neuroretinal rim area and volume, as well as cup area and volume.

Although previous versions of OCT technology (TD-OCT) were also able to provide such measurements, a large amount of data interpolation was required, resulting in poor reproducibility and accuracy of the measurements. The improved resolution and velocity of scan acquisition of SD-OCT have greatly reduced the need for interpolation,

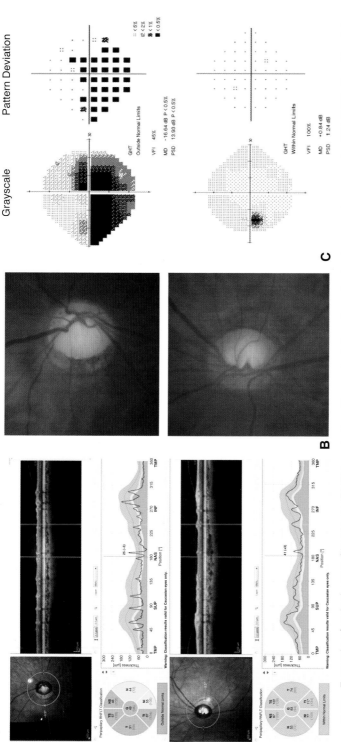

Figure 3-18 Example of retinal nerve fiber layer (RNFL) analysis with spectral-domain optical coherence tomography (SD-OCT). *Top:* The right eye shows diffuse RNFL thinning on SD-OCT **(A)**, which is consistent with the neuroretinal rim thinning and enlarged cup seen in the photographs of the optic nerve head **(B)** and with the visual field loss that is evident on standard automated perimetry (SAP) **(C)**. *Bottom:* The left eye shows normal RNFL thickness on SD-OCT **(A)**, normal appearance of the optic nerve head **(B)**, and normal visual field **(C)**. *(Courtesy of Felipe A. Medeiros, MD, PhD.)*

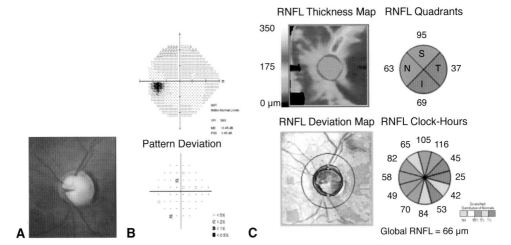

Figure 3-19 **A,** Photograph of the optic nerve head shows marked neuroretinal rim thinning and an enlarged cup; however, SAP **(B)** shows that the visual field is still within normal limits. **C,** The RNFL analysis with SD-OCT shows diffuse loss of the RNFL. *(Courtesy of Felipe A. Medeiros, MD, PhD.)*

resulting in much better delineation of optic nerve head structures. Figure 3-20 shows measurements obtained from different scanning areas (RNFL, optic nerve head, and macula) with SD-OCT.

Confocal scanning laser ophthalmoscopy is another technology that can be used for assessing glaucomatous damage to the optic nerve head. The optical design of instruments using confocal scanning laser technology allows for a series of tomographic slices, or optical sections, of the structure being imaged. Parameters such as cup area, cup volume, rim volume, cup–disc ratio, and peripapillary nerve fiber layer thickness are then calculated based on the location of the vitreoretinal interface.

The *scanning laser polarimeter* is a scanning laser ophthalmoscope outfitted with a polarization modulator and detector to take advantage of the birefringent properties of the RNFL in order to estimate its thickness. The birefringence of the RNFL arises from the predominantly parallel nature of the axonal microtubule substructure. As light passes through the nerve fiber layer, the polarization state changes. The deeper layers of retinal tissue reflect the light back to the detector, where the degree to which the polarization has been changed is recorded. The fundamental parameter being measured with this instrumentation is *relative* (not absolute) RNFL thickness. The addition of a variable corneal compensator and an enhanced corneal compensator to include analysis of potential anterior segment birefringence has improved the quality of the information available with this technique.

Although imaging devices are largely used as ancillary tests aimed at detecting early signs of glaucomatous damage, perhaps their greatest value is in the longitudinal monitoring of structural damage by serial imaging over time. Several investigations have shown that imaging parameters, such as RNFL thickness or rim area, are able to detect progressive glaucomatous damage. In addition, these parameters can provide quantitative assessment of rates of change in the disease, which are essential in establishing appropriate treatment (Fig 3-21). Although most glaucoma patients will show some evidence

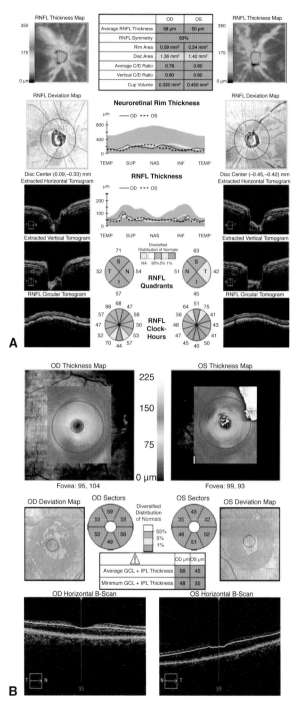

Figure 3-20 SD-OCT analysis of different regions of a glaucomatous eye. **A,** The printout shows RNFL and optic nerve head analyses. Several parameters are provided, including average RNFL thickness, rim area, disc area, and cup–disc (C/D) ratio. **B,** The printout shows analysis of the macular area, with the parameter ganglion cell layer + inner plexiform layer (GCL+IPL) thickness. *(Courtesy of Felipe A. Medeiros, MD, PhD.)*

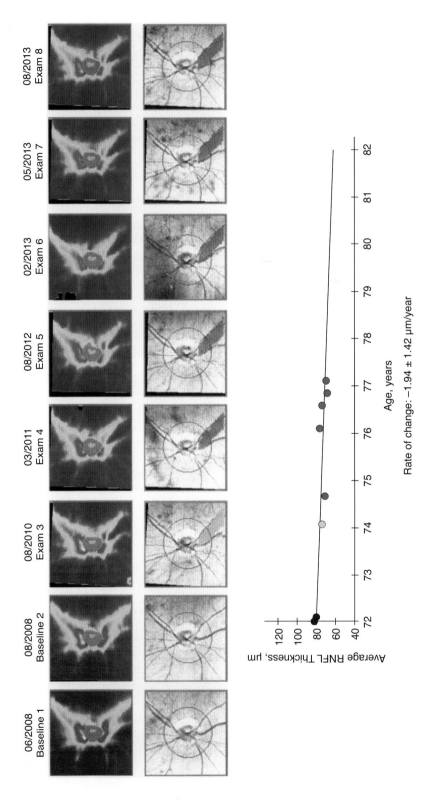

Figure 3-21 SD-OCT images showing progressive RNFL loss. There is progressive loss of the RNFL in the inferotemporal sector. The plot at the bottom of the figure shows the rate of change in the parameter average RNFL thickness. *(Courtesy of Felipe A. Medeiros, MD, PhD.)*

of progression if followed long enough, the rate of deterioration can be highly variable among them. While most patients progress relatively slowly, others have aggressive disease with fast deterioration, which can eventually result in blindness or substantial impairment unless appropriate interventions take place. Importantly, progressive structural damage may occur despite lack of detectable visual field deterioration. These structural changes, however, have been shown to predict future functional deterioration in glaucoma patients. Therefore, comprehensive assessment of glaucomatous damage should involve both structural and functional evaluations.

Lisboa R, Leite MT, Zangwill LM, Tafreshi A, Weinreb RN, Medeiros FA. Diagnosing pre-perimetric glaucoma with spectral domain optical coherence tomography. *Ophthalmology.* 2012;119(11):2261–2269.

The Visual Field

For many years, the standard method of measuring the visual dysfunction seen with glaucomatous injury has been assessment of the visual field with clinical *perimetry,* which measures differential light sensitivity, or the ability of the subject to distinguish a stimulus from a uniform background.

Perimetry has traditionally served 2 major purposes in the management of glaucoma:

1. identification and quantification of abnormal fields
2. longitudinal assessment to detect glaucomatous progression and measure rates of change

Quantification of visual field sensitivity enables detection of visual field defects by comparison with normative data. Regular visual field testing in known cases of disease provides valuable information for helping to differentiate between stability and progressive loss.

Automated static perimetry is currently the standard method for assessing visual function in glaucoma. With this method, threshold sensitivity measurements are usually performed at a number of test locations using white stimuli on a white background; this is known as *standard automated perimetry (SAP),* or achromatic automated perimetry. Automated static perimetry has largely replaced manual kinetic perimetry, which is now rarely performed for visual field assessment in glaucoma. However, manual kinetic perimetry may be helpful for monitoring visual fields in patients who are unable to perform the automated test.

Factors Affecting Perimetry Results

Many factors may affect the results obtained from perimetry, including the patient's level of attentiveness, the perimetrist's administration of the test, and other variables, such as refractive correction. The interaction between the perimetrist and the patient is fundamental to enhance the chances of successful perimetric testing.

Patient

People vary in their attentiveness and response time from moment to moment and from day to day. Longer tests are more likely to produce fatigue and diminish the ability of the patient to maintain peak performance.

Perimetrist

Although the influence of the perimetrist on the results of automated perimetry is in general smaller than with manual perimetry, the perimetrist still plays a fundamental role in the outcome of the test. It is important to instruct the patient about what to expect during the test, such as how long the test will take, when to blink, what the stimulus will look like, and where it might appear. Also, it is important to advise patients that the stimuli are likely to be barely visible throughout the test, and that more than half of the stimuli shown in a threshold test will not be visible. This can decrease a patient's anxiety and improve cooperation during the test. In addition, the perimetrist should explain to the patient how he or she could pause the test if necessary. The patient should be monitored during the test, to ensure proper positioning and fixation, and the perimetrist should be available to intervene if necessary to ensure proper testing conditions.

Other factors

Several other factors may affect the results of perimetry, including background luminance, stimulus luminance, and size of the stimulus. In automated perimetry, these variables are standardized according to the specific testing strategy being employed, allowing reliable comparisons of tests obtained with the same strategy over time.

Other factors that may affect perimetry results include patient refraction and pupil size. Uncorrected refractive errors cause blurring on the retina and decrease the visibility of stimuli. Thus, proper neutralization of refractive errors is essential for accurate perimetry. In addition, presbyopic patients must have a refractive compensation that focuses fixation at the depth of the perimeter bowl. Care needs to be taken to center the patient close to the correcting lens to avoid a lens rim artifact. A small pupil (<2.5 mm) may produce artifacts on perimetry by reducing the amount of light entering the eye. However, such artifacts are now rare because of the less common use of miotics.

Automated Static Perimetry

A computerized perimeter must be able to determine differential light sensitivity at multiple points in the retina, to perform an adequate test in a reasonable amount of time, and to present results in a comprehensible form. Various strategies have been used in order to obtain reliable and efficient estimates of threshold visual sensitivity in perimetry.

With the Humphrey Field Analyzer (HFA) perimeter (Carl-Zeiss Meditec, Dublin, CA), the Swedish interactive threshold algorithm (SITA) has largely replaced the older full-threshold strategy as the standard method for threshold measurement. SITA is a Bayesian test strategy that uses prior information from previous evaluations of healthy individuals and persons with disease to generate a probability distribution function (PDF) representing the probabilities that the visual field sensitivity will be of a particular value at a particular visual field location. As the test progresses, the distribution is then adjusted, according to whether or not the person being tested responds to the stimulus presentations. This continues until the PDF distribution is within a small range, at which point the mean of the distribution is selected as the threshold sensitivity estimate. The PDFs are adjusted for the age of the individual, the visual field location tested, the sensitivity values of neighboring test locations, and the results of previous stimulus presentations. SITA has been demonstrated to have equal or lower test–retest variability compared with conventional staircase procedures employed in the older full-threshold strategy, and testing can often be done in half the time.

The SITA strategy is available in the Humphrey perimeters as SITA Standard and SITA Fast. SITA Standard is usually the strategy of choice. SITA Fast is even faster than SITA Standard and may have similar accuracy and reliability; however, it may be a more difficult test for the patient because the test stimuli tend to be closer to the patient's threshold, thus offering less positive feedback to the patient. Patients who are perceived to have difficulties with SITA Standard should not be shifted to SITA Fast; they should continue with SITA Standard. These patients will generally benefit from careful instruction by the perimetrist, closer surveillance, and positive feedback.

Similar to the SITA test strategy for the HFA, the *tendency-oriented perimeter (TOP)* algorithm was developed for the Octopus perimeter (Haag-Streit, Mason, OH) as an alternative to the lengthy staircase threshold procedures. However, TOP is distinct from SITA in that only 1 stimulus is shown at a single location of the visual field. Therefore, in order to estimate the threshold sensitivity at a particular location, TOP supplements this single data point per test location with information obtained at adjoining test locations.

Threshold tests

The most common programs for glaucoma testing are the central 24° and 30° programs, such as the Octopus 32 and G1 and the Humphrey 24-2 and 30-2 (Fig 3-22). These programs test the central field using a 6° grid. They test points 3° above and 3° below the horizontal midline and facilitate diagnosis of defects that respect this line. A 24-2 test

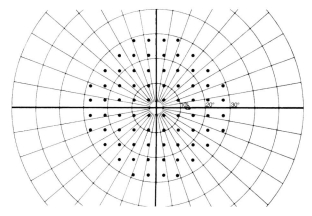

Figure 3-22 Central 30-2 threshold test pattern, right eye. *(Reproduced with permission from* The Field Analyzer Primer. *San Leandro, CA: Allergan Humphrey; 1989.)*

performed with the SITA Standard strategy for obtaining threshold estimates is then usually referred to as *SITA Standard 24-2*. For patients with advanced visual field loss or with paracentral defects, serial 10-2 or C8 visual field testing should also be used (Fig 3-23). These visual fields concentrate on the central 8°–10° of the visual field, and test points every 1°–2°, enabling the ophthalmologist to follow many more test points within the central island and improve detection of progression. Alternatively, a larger stimulus (Size V) can be used in more advanced patients.

Although a 30°–60° program is available on most static threshold perimeters, it is rarely performed because the threshold variability is very high in these more peripheral regions.

Screening tests

These tests may or may not be threshold-related, and they cover varying areas of the visual field. Suprathreshold tests are not recommended for glaucoma suspects because they do not provide a good reference for future comparison. They may be useful with other conditions causing visual field loss, however.

Interpretation of a Single Visual Field

The clinician should exercise caution when interpreting perimetric results. Even with improved strategies, these remain subjective tests. Therefore, confirmation of a new defect or worsening of an existing defect is usually necessary to validate the clinical implication of the visual field in conjunction with all other pertinent data. Evaluation of the visual field involves (1) assessing the quality or reliability of the visual field test, (2) assessing the normality or abnormality, and (3) identifying artifacts.

Quality

The first aspect of the field to be evaluated is its quality or reliability. Reliability indices include the percentage of fixation losses, false-positives and false-negatives. Of these, a high percentage of false-positives is most detrimental to a visual field test. The false-positive rate measures the tendency of the patient to press the response button even when no stimulus has been seen. Visual fields with a false-positive rate greater than 15% are likely unreliable and nonrepresentative of the patient's true field status. A high fixation loss rate (>25%) is also indicative of an unreliable field, especially if accompanied by the lack of a well-demarcated blind spot. False-negative rates measure the tendency of the patient to fail to press the button even when a visible stimulus has been presented. Although a high false-negative rate could indicate an inattentive patient, damaged areas of the visual field show increased variability, which can lead to a high false-negative rate. Therefore, although the percentage of false-negatives has also traditionally been included as a reliability index, false-negative rates can be elevated in abnormal fields regardless of the attentiveness of the patient. Hence, visual field tests should not necessarily be disregarded because of high false-negative rates.

Normality or abnormality

The next aspect of the visual field to be assessed is its normality or abnormality. When tested under photopic conditions, the normal visual field demonstrates the greatest

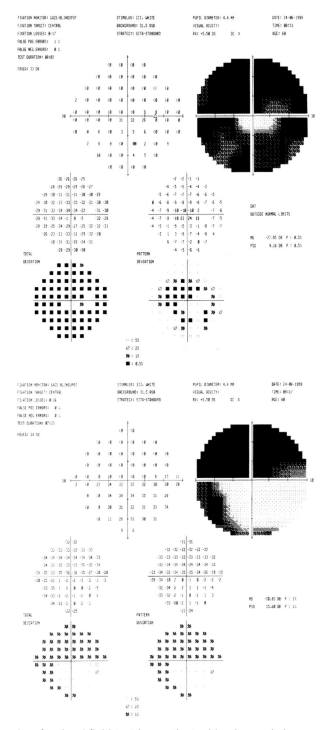

Figure 3-23 Results of a visual field test in a patient with advanced glaucomatous visual field loss. The test with 30-2 pattern *(top)* evaluates only a few points in the central area. The 10-2 test *(bottom)* evaluates more points in the central area, allowing better evaluation of potential progression over time in this case. *(Courtesy of Felipe A. Medeiros, MD, PhD.)*

sensitivity centrally, with sensitivity falling steadily toward the periphery. Figure 3-24 shows a single field analysis of a visual field obtained with the Humphrey perimeter. The results are presented as a series of numerical plots and probability maps including a threshold sensitivity map with the numerical threshold sensitivities for each location and

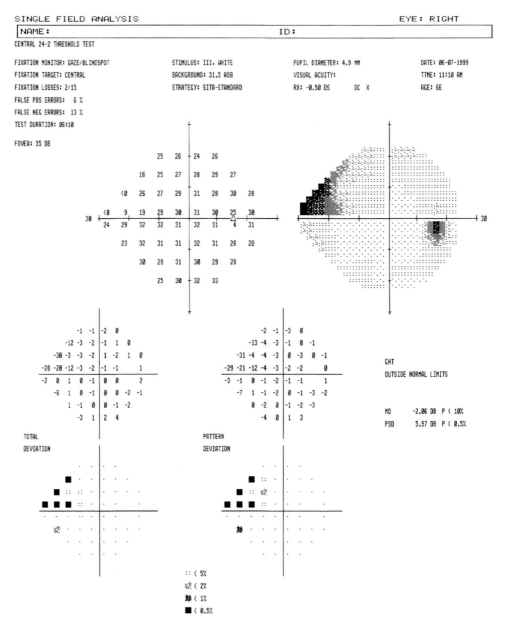

Figure 3-24 Printout of a visual field test obtained with a Humphrey field analyzer using the SITA Standard 24-2 test.

a corresponding grayscale map; a total deviation plot, showing decibel deviations from age-corrected normal sensitivities; a total deviation probability map, showing deviations that fall outside the statistical range of normal sensitivity; a pattern deviation map, showing the localized loss after correcting for overall decreases in sensitivity; and a pattern deviation probability map.

The Humphrey perimeter also provides a series of summary indices, including Mean Deviation (MD), which is a weighted average of the total deviation values, where zero equates to no deviation from normal and more negative values indicate more advanced loss; Pattern Standard Deviation (PSD), which is a summary index of localized visual field loss; and the Glaucoma Hemifield Test (GHT), which categorizes eyes as within normal limits, borderline, or outside normal limits based on a comparison of visual field sensitivities at corresponding areas of the superior and inferior hemifields. As glaucoma frequently causes asymmetric damage to the superior and inferior hemifields, the GHT offers a powerful tool for identification of glaucomatous visual field defects (Fig 3-25).

Several criteria have been proposed for identification of visual field abnormalities. A simple and widely accepted criterion is the one employed by the Ocular Hypertension Treatment Study (OHTS). In the OHTS, a visual field defect was defined as the presence of a PSD with P <5% or the presence of a GHT with a result outside normal limits. The abnormality had to be present in 3 consecutive visual field tests. In the analysis of a visual field printout, it is also important to evaluate the probability maps, especially the pattern deviation probability plot. The presence of a cluster of at least 3 abnormal points (P <5%) on the pattern deviation plot, with at least 1 of those points with P <1%, has also been used as criterion for visual field defect.

It is important to emphasize that the clinician should examine the visual fields to verify whether the defect is repeatable and present in approximately the same location, and that the abnormalities are not due to the presence of artifacts. Although the points that are abnormal will not be exactly the same in all confirmatory tests, the area of visual field abnormality should be similar among the tests.

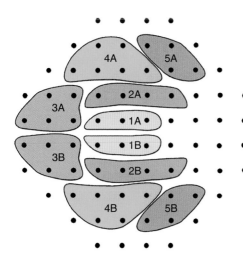

Figure 3-25 The Glaucoma Hemifield Test compares pattern deviation probability values in 5 predetermined zones in the superior hemifield with corresponding zones in the inferior hemifield. *(Reproduced with permission from Heijl A, Bengtsson B, Patella VM. Effective Perimetry. 4th ed. Jena, Germany: Carl Zeiss Meditec AG; 2012:53.)*

Artifacts

Identification of artifacts is the next step in evaluation of the visual field. The following are common artifacts seen on automated perimetry:

- *Lens rim:* If the patient's corrective lens is decentered or set too far from the eye, the lens rim may project into the central 30° (Fig 3-26).
- *Incorrect corrective lens:* If an incorrect corrective lens is used, the resulting field will be generally depressed.
- *Eyelid artifact:* Partial eyelid ptosis may lead to an artifactual superior visual field defect.
- *Cloverleaf visual field:* If a patient stops paying attention and ceases to respond partway through a visual field test, a distinctive visual field pattern may develop. Figure 3-27 shows a cloverleaf visual field, the result of the testing order of the Humphrey 30-2 perimeter, which begins testing with the points circled in this figure and proceeds outward. This pattern may also be seen if a patient is malingering.

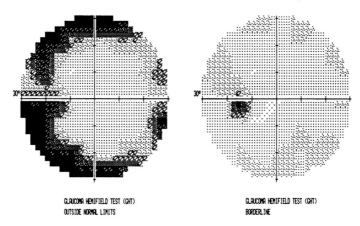

GLAUCOMA HEMIFIELD TEST (GHT)
OUTSIDE NORMAL LIMITS

GLAUCOMA HEMIFIELD TEST (GHT)
BORDERLINE

Figure 3-26 Lens rim artifact. The 2 visual fields shown were obtained 9 days apart. The visual field on the left shows a typical lens rim artifact, whereas the corrective lens was positioned appropriately for the visual field on the right (Humphrey 30-2 program).

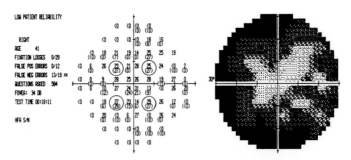

Figure 3-27 Cloverleaf visual field. The Humphrey visual field perimeter test is designed so that 4 circled points are checked initially and the testing in each quadrant proceeds outward from these points. If the patient ceases to respond after only a few points have been tested, the result is some variation of the cloverleaf visual field shown at right (Humphrey 30-2 program).

- *High false-positive rate:* When a patient responds at a time when no test stimulus is being presented, a false-positive response is recorded. False-positive rates greater than 15% suggest an unreliable test that can mask or minimize an actual scotoma and can, in extreme cases, result in a visual field with impossibly high threshold values (Fig 3-28). Careful instruction of the patient may sometimes resolve this artifact.

Patterns of Visual Field Loss in Glaucoma

The hallmark defect of glaucoma is the nerve fiber bundle defect that results from damage at the optic nerve head. The pattern of nerve fibers in the retinal area served by the

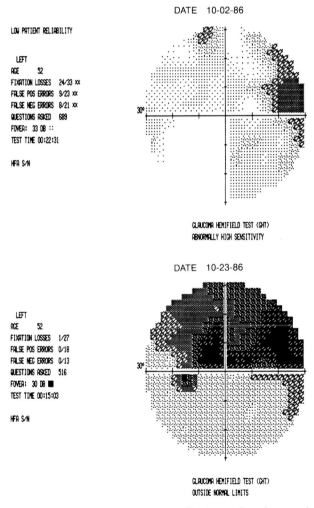

Figure 3-28 High false-positive rate. The top visual field contains characteristic "white scotomata," which represent areas of impossibly high retinal sensitivity. On the return visit 3 weeks later, the patient was carefully instructed to respond only when she saw the light, resulting in the bottom visual field, which shows good reliability and demonstrates the patient's dense superior visual field loss (Humphrey 30-2 program).

damaged nerve fiber bundle will correspond to the specific defect. The common names for the classic visual field defects are derived from their appearance as plotted on a kinetic visual field chart. In static perimetry, however, the sample points are in a grid pattern, and the representation of visual field defects on a static perimetry chart generally lacks the smooth contours suggested by such terms as *arcuate.*

Glaucomatous visual field defects include the following:

- arcuate or Bjerrum scotoma (Fig 3-29)
- nasal step (Fig 3-30)
- paracentral scotoma (Fig 3-31)

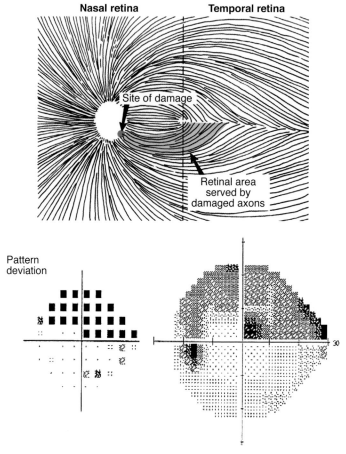

Figure 3-29 An *arcuate scotoma* occurs in the area 10°–20° from fixation. Glaucomatous damage to a nerve fiber bundle containing axons from both the inferonasal and inferotemporal retina resulted in the arcuate defect shown. The scotoma often begins as a single area of relative loss, which then becomes larger, deeper, and multifocal. In its full form, an arcuate scotoma arches from the blind spot and ends at the nasal raphe, becoming wider and closer to fixation on the nasal side (Humphrey 24-2 program). *(Visual field courtesy of G. A. Cioffi, MD.)*

- altitudinal defect (Fig 3-32)
- generalized depression (rare in glaucoma in the absence of localized loss)
- temporal wedge (rare)

The superior and inferior poles of the optic nerve appear to be most susceptible to glaucomatous damage. However, damage to small, scattered bundles of optic nerve axons commonly produces a generalized decrease in sensitivity, which is harder to recognize than focal defects. Combinations of superior and inferior visual field loss, such as double arcuate scotomata, may occur, resulting in profound peripheral vision loss. Typically, the central island of vision and the inferotemporal visual field are retained until late in the course of glaucomatous optic nerve damage (see Fig 3-23).

Heijl A, Bengtsson B, Patella VM. *Effective Perimetry.* 4th ed. Jena, Germany: Carl Zeiss Meditec AG; 2012.

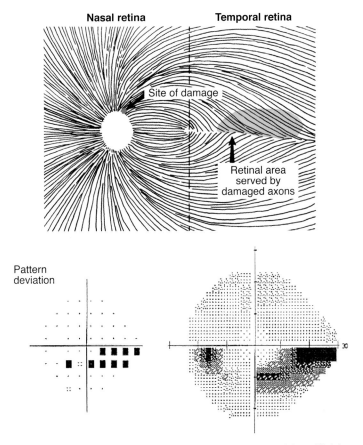

Figure 3-30 A *nasal step* is a relative depression of one horizontal hemifield compared with the other. Damage to superior nerve fibers serving the superotemporal retina beyond the paracentral area resulted in this nasal step. In kinetic perimetry, the nasal step is defined as a discontinuity or depression in one or more nasal isopters near the horizontal raphe (Humphrey 24-2 program). *(Visual field courtesy of G. A. Cioffi, MD.)*

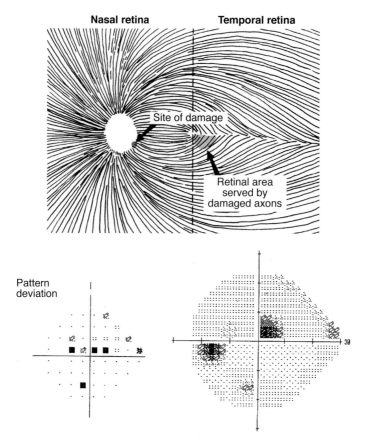

Figure 3-31 A *paracentral scotoma* is an island of relative or absolute vision loss within 10° of fixation. Loss of nerve fibers from the inferior pole, originating from the inferotemporal retina, resulted in the superonasal scotoma shown. Paracentral scotomata may be single, as in this case, or multiple, and they may occur as isolated findings or may be associated with other early defects (Humphrey 24-2 program). *(Visual field courtesy of G. A. Cioffi, MD.)*

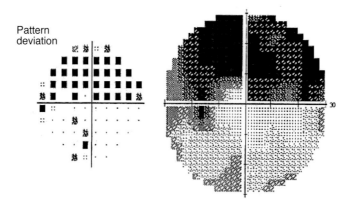

Figure 3-32 Altitudinal defect with nearly complete loss of the superior visual field, characteristic of moderate to advanced glaucomatous optic neuropathy (left eye). *(Visual field courtesy of G. A. Cioffi, MD.)*

Interpretation of a Series of Visual Fields and Detection of Visual Field Progression

Interpretation of serial visual fields should meet 2 goals:

1. separating real change from ordinary variation
2. using the information obtained from visual field testing to determine the likelihood that a change is related to glaucomatous progression

Visual field testing is a subjective examination, and different responses may be obtained each time the test is performed or even during the same test. This fluctuation can greatly confound the interpretation of change. In order to detect true visual field progression, one needs to evaluate whether the observed change exceeds the expected variability for a particular area.

There are, in general, 2 main approaches to analyzing visual field progression. The first approach is to compare the results of the current examination with those from a previous one (usually set as the baseline). If the results of the follow-up examination are significantly worse, progression is indicated. This approach is called *event-based analysis,* as it looks for defects on the current examination that were not present before.

In the second approach, instead of comparing the current test with a baseline test, one looks for progressive change by analyzing all the tests available in a specific period. This is called *trend-based analysis,* as change is observed as a trend in the values plotted over time, and significant deterioration can be assessed by observing the slope or decline of the regression line. In addition to evaluating whether progression has occurred, trend analysis allows estimation of the rate of progression. It is well known that some patients decline faster than others, and estimating each individual's rate of progression is helpful for predicting the risk of functional impairment and determining how aggressive the treatment should be.

Different tools are available to assist clinicians in identifying visual field progression, and there is no consensus about the best method for detecting change. The simplest and most general method uses the Mean Deviation (MD) index plotted against time. A statistically significant decline would indicate progressive deterioration. Deterioration on the MD index may represent glaucomatous progression or progression of cataract or other media opacities. Conversely, in a glaucoma patient who has undergone cataract surgery, progression may be masked in evaluation by this method.

The Humphrey perimeter provides Guided Progression Analysis (GPA) software to assist in detection of visual field progression (Fig 3-33). The software presents an event-based method that is based on the pattern deviation plot and, therefore, adjusts for the potential confounding effects of diffuse loss of sensitivity from media opacities. Detection of new or progressing visual field defects is performed by comparison to the baseline; therefore, it is critical to have reliable baseline examinations. Often, the patient experiences a learning effect, and the second visual field may show substantial improvement over the first. At least 2 visual field tests should be performed as early as possible in the course of a patient's disease. If the results are quite different, a third test should be performed. The software automatically selects the first 2 available examinations as the baseline tests. However, one can easily override this selection to a more suitable time-point (eg, change in therapy after progression), or to avoid initial learning effects (which could reduce the sensitivity to detect progression). The software then compares each follow-up test to

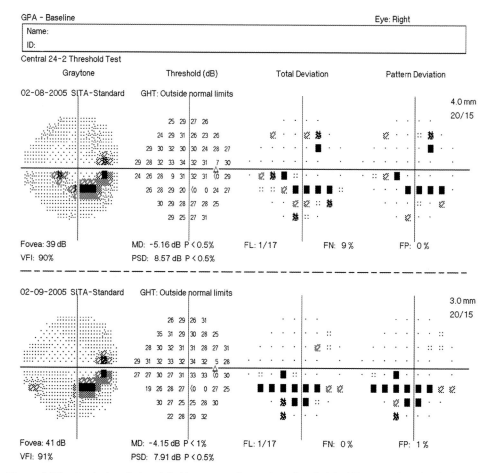

Figure 3-33 Analysis of visual field progression using the Guided Progression Analysis software of the Humphrey perimeter. These visual fields were selected as the baseline. Results of each follow-up visual field test (see Fig 3-34) are compared with the average of the 2 baseline fields. *(Courtesy of Felipe A. Medeiros, MD, PhD.)*

the average of the baseline tests (Fig 3-34). It identifies points that show change greater than the expected variability (at the 95% significance level), as determined by previous studies with stable glaucoma patients. If significant change is detected in at least 3 points and repeated in the same points in 2 consecutive follow-up tests, the software will flag the last examination as *Possible Progression.* If significant change is detected and repeated for the same 3 or more points in 3 consecutive follow-up tests, the GPA software will flag the last examination as *Likely Progression.*

The most recent version of the GPA software also provides the Visual Field Index (VFI) and VFI progression plot (Fig 3-35). The VFI is designed to better evaluate the rate of progression with SAP. The VFI is calculated as the percentage of normal visual field, after adjustment for age. Therefore, a VFI of 100% represents a completely normal visual field, while a VFI of 0% represents a perimetrically blind visual field. The VFI is shown on the GPA printout both as a percentage value for each examination and as a trend analysis,

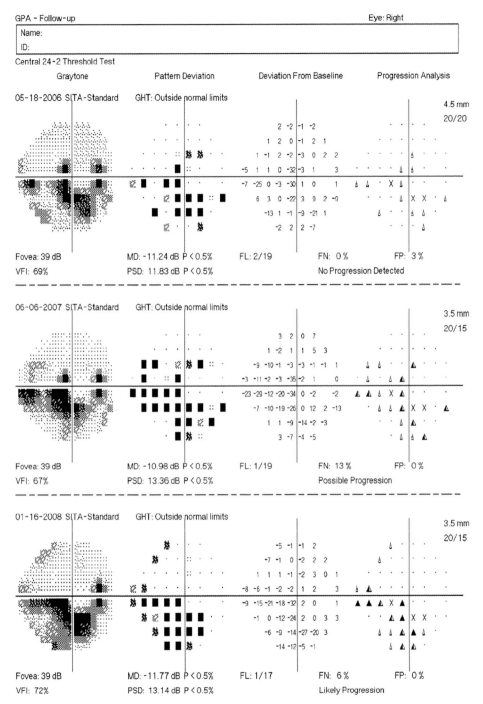

Figure 3-34 Visual fields from consecutive follow-up examinations (see Fig 3-33 for baseline visual field tests for this patient). Several points are flagged as showing significant deterioration. A number of points in the inferonasal region show repeatable significant change *(black-filled triangles)*. The last visual field is then flagged as Likely Progression. *(Courtesy of Felipe A. Medeiros, MD, PhD.)*

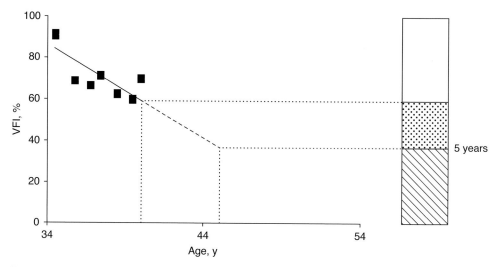

Rate of progression: −4.5 ± 3.3%/year (95% CI)
Slope significant at $P < 5\%$

Figure 3-35 Humphrey Visual Field Index (VFI) plot corresponding to the visual fields shown in Figures 3-33 and 3-34. The slope of change was significant and estimated at −4.5% per year. CI = confidence interval. *(Courtesy of Felipe A. Medeiros, MD, PhD.)*

plotted against age. While the MD is based only on the total deviation map, and thus largely affected by cataract, the VFI is based both on the pattern deviation probability map, for the identification of possibly progressing points, and on the total deviation map, used for the actual calculation of change of the total deviation value. In addition, the algorithm uses different weights for different locations, giving more weight to more central points, which have higher impact on the patient's quality of vision. The final VFI score is the mean of all weighted scores.

The Octopus perimeter also provides a comprehensive statistical package (EyeSuite) for evaluation of visual field progression. The software calculates rates of progression in terms of mean defect change per year (in dB/year), similar to the MD index from Humphrey perimetry. In addition, the software provides an analysis of progression by individual test points (pointwise linear regression) and by clusters, where test locations are combined according to nerve fiber bundle patterns.

> Bengtsson B, Heijl A. A visual field index for calculation of glaucoma rate of progression. *Am J Ophthalmol.* 2008;145(2):343–353.

Structure and function correlations

It is important to correlate changes in the visual field with those in the optic nerve head. If such correlation is lacking, the ophthalmologist should consider other causes of vision loss, such as ischemic optic neuropathy, demyelinating or other neurologic disease, or pituitary tumor. This consideration is especially important in the following situations:

- The patient's optic nerve head seems less cupped than would be expected for the degree of visual field loss.
- The pallor of the optic nerve head is more impressive than the cupping.

- The progression of the visual field loss seems excessive.
- The pattern of visual field loss is uncharacteristic for glaucoma—for example, it respects the vertical midline.
- The location of the cupping or thinning of the neural rim does not correspond to the proper location of the visual field defect.

It should be noted, however, that progressive visual field loss may sometimes be seen in the absence of optic nerve head changes and vice versa. In cases of early disease, progressive structural changes to the optic nerve and RNFL can frequently be seen despite lack of apparent visual field progression. Conversely, in cases of more severe disease, progressive visual field losses tend to occur despite lack of detectable structural change. This apparent disagreement may be explained by the different characteristics of the tests, including scaling, variability, and presence of floor/ceiling effects. Therefore, follow-up of glaucoma patients should be performed using both structural and functional assessments.

Medeiros FA, Zangwill LM, Bowd C, Mansouri K, Weinreb RN. The structure and function relationship in glaucoma: implications for detection of progression and measurement of rates of change. *Invest Ophthalmol Vis Sci.* 2012;53(11):6939–6946.

Other Perimetric Tests

Other psychophysical tests of visual function have been developed, including frequency-doubling technology (FDT), short-wavelength automated perimetry (SWAP), and flicker-defined form (FDF) perimetry (Fig 3-36). These tests aim to target subpopulations of retinal ganglion cells (RGCs) by evaluating specific aspects of visual function (eg, motion perception, contrast sensitivity, color vision) and thereby reduce the ability of the visual system to use other pathways to compensate. It has been hypothesized that in its early stages, glaucoma may predominately damage magnocellular RGCs projecting to the magnocellular layers of the lateral geniculate nucleus (ie, the magnocellular [M] pathway).

FDT perimetry, which determines the contrast sensitivity for detecting a high temporal frequency counter-phase flicker stimulus, was designed to selectively evaluate the M pathway; evidence shows that the response to motion perimetry may be generated by many ganglion cell types and is cortically mediated. Nevertheless, FDT has shown promise for glaucoma detection, and longitudinal studies have shown that abnormalities on FDT may precede detectable SAP changes in many patients.

SWAP uses a narrow band blue-violet stimulus (440-nm wavelength) against a bright yellow background illumination. SWAP targets the small bistratified ganglion cells, which project their axons to the koniocellular layers of the lateral geniculate nucleus. SWAP has also been modified over the years and now utilizes the SITA strategy to shorten the test duration. Despite these modifications, however, SWAP SITA generally does not have better diagnostic ability than SAP and is now rarely performed in clinical practice.

The FDF stimulus has been proposed as an alternative method for detecting glaucomatous vision loss. FDF perimetry is believed to stimulate the M pathway, and there is emerging evidence that it may be useful for early glaucoma diagnosis.

Although psychophysical tests such as FDT, SWAP, and FDF perimetry attempt to minimize potential input from other pathways, it is unlikely any stimulus can be 100% specific for a single visual pathway or a single subset of RGCs. Furthermore, there is not a

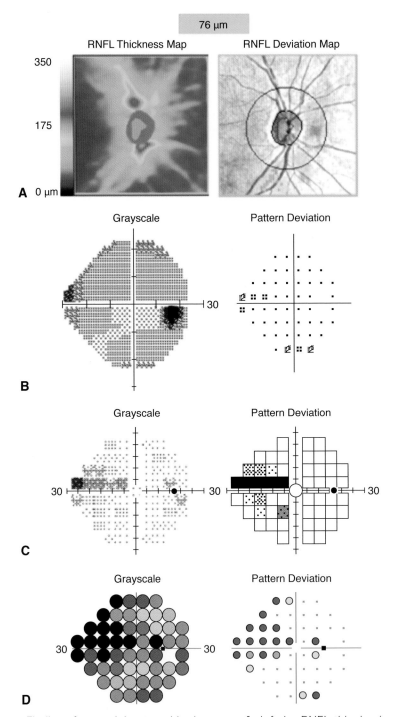

Figure 3-36 Findings from a right eye with glaucoma. **A,** Inferior RNFL thinning is visible on OCT. **B,** SAP shows a small corresponding superonasal visual field defect that is more pronounced on frequency-doubling technology perimetry **(C)** and Heidelberg Edge Perimetry **(D).** *(Courtesy of Felipe A. Medeiros, MD, PhD.)*

single ganglion cell type that is always affected first in glaucoma. Perimetric tests are also subjective examinations and therefore responses may vary on repeat testing, or during the same test, reducing the ability to confidently detect genuine early abnormalities.

Other tests measuring the integrity of the visual field include contrast sensitivity perimetry, flicker sensitivity, microperimetry, visually evoked cortical potential, and multifocal electroretinography. However, these tests are not commonly employed in the evaluation of patients with glaucoma. Several of these tests are discussed in greater detail in BCSC Section 12, *Retina and Vitreous*.

Meira-Freitas D, Tatham AJ, Lisboa R, et al. Predicting progression of glaucoma from rates of frequency doubling technology perimetry change. *Ophthalmology.* 2014;121(2):498–507.

Other Tests for Selected Patients

Several other tests may be helpful in selected patients. Many of these tests are described elsewhere in the BCSC series, and the reader is advised to consult the *Master Index* for the following:

- fluorescein angiography
- corneal pachymetry
- corneal hysteresis
- measurement of episcleral venous pressure
- carotid noninvasive vascular studies
- ocular blood-flow measurements
- ultrasonography

Ultrasound biomicroscopy (UBM) may provide information about anterior segment anatomy in several types of glaucoma. The test employs shorter-wavelength sound waves than does conventional ocular ultrasonography, limiting penetration through the sclera but increasing the resolution. UBM allows detailed examination of the anterior segment, the posterior chamber, and the ciliary body. Anterior segment optical coherence tomography (AS-OCT) may also provide images of the anterior segment and angle. However, although the resolution of AS-OCT is better than that of UBM, penetration through the sclera is minimal with AS-OCT, reducing its ability to provide images of the ciliary body and adjacent structures.

CHAPTER 4

Open-Angle Glaucoma

Primary Open-Angle Glaucoma

Primary open-angle glaucoma (POAG) is typically a chronic, slowly progressive optic neuropathy with characteristic patterns of optic nerve damage and visual field loss. Numerous clinical factors affect an individual's susceptibility to POAG, which is a multifactorial disease process. These include elevated intraocular pressure (IOP), advanced age, race, thin central cornea, and a positive family history of glaucoma. Other factors that may contribute to disease susceptibility include corneal hysteresis, low ocular perfusion pressure, low cerebrospinal fluid pressure, abnormalities of axonal or ganglion cell metabolism, and disorders of the extracellular matrix of the lamina cribrosa. Unfortunately, we do not yet fully understand the interplay of the multiple factors involved in the development of POAG. *Secondary* OAG differs from POAG in that identifiable factors contribute to its development, such as pigment dispersion in pigmentary glaucoma and the pseudoexfoliative material of pseudoexfoliation syndrome.

Clinical Features

POAG is typically insidious in onset, slowly progressive, and painless. It is usually bilateral but can be quite asymmetric. Patients may seem relatively asymptomatic until the later stages of the disease, when central vision is affected. POAG is diagnosed based on findings from the assessment of the optic nerve and nerve fiber layer and the results of visual field testing.

Gonioscopic findings

To establish a diagnosis of POAG, the clinician must verify that the anterior chamber angle is open. Gonioscopy (discussed in Chapter 3) should be performed on all patients evaluated for glaucoma and should be repeated periodically in patients with established OAG to monitor for progressive angle closure caused by lens-induced changes, particularly in patients with hyperopia. Repeated gonioscopy is also indicated when the chamber becomes shallow; when strong miotics are prescribed; after argon laser trabeculoplasty or laser peripheral iridotomy has been performed; or when IOP increases.

Optic nerve head appearance and visual fields

Although elevated IOP is an important risk factor for OAG, diagnosis of this disease is based primarily on the appearance of the optic nerve head, or optic disc, and on the results of visual field testing. See Chapter 3 for a detailed discussion of the optic nerve head and visual fields. Careful periodic evaluation of the optic nerve and visual field testing are essential in the management of glaucoma. Stereophotographic documentation of the optic nerve or computerized imaging of the optic nerve or retinal nerve fiber layer aids the detection of subtle changes over time. Visual field loss should correlate with the appearance of the optic nerve; significant discrepancies between the pattern of visual field loss and optic nerve appearance warrant additional investigation, as noted in Chapter 3.

American Academy of Ophthalmology Glaucoma Panel. Preferred Practice Pattern Guidelines. *Primary Open-Angle Glaucoma.* San Francisco: American Academy of Ophthalmology; 2010. Available at www.aao.org/ppp.

Jonas JB, Budde WM, Panda-Jonas S. Ophthalmoscopic evaluation of the optic nerve head. *Surv Ophthalmol.* 1999;43(4):293–320.

Risk Factors

Intraocular pressure

Elevated IOP is an important risk factor for glaucoma, but it is not required for a diagnosis of POAG. While large population-based studies suggest a mean IOP of 15.5 mm Hg (standard deviation ±2.6) in European-derived populations, the normal distribution of IOP varies across racial and ethnic groups. This conclusion led to the definition of "normal" IOP as 2 standard deviations above and below the mean IOP, or ranging between 10 and 21 mm Hg. IOP greater than 21 mm Hg was thus traditionally defined as "abnormal." However, this definition has a number of shortcomings.

It is known that IOP in the general population is not represented by a Gaussian distribution but rather is skewed toward higher pressures (see Chapter 2, Fig 2-4). Thus, IOPs of 22 mm Hg and above may not necessarily be abnormal from a statistical standpoint. More importantly, IOP distribution curves for glaucomatous and nonglaucomatous eyes show a great deal of overlap. Several studies indicate that as many as 30%–50% of individuals in the general population with glaucomatous optic neuropathy and/or visual field loss have initial IOP measurements below 22 mm Hg. Elevations of IOP may occur only intermittently in some glaucomatous eyes, with as many as one-third of these elevated measurements due to normal circadian fluctuation.

In patients with glaucoma, IOP may vary considerably—by 10 mm Hg or more—over a 24-hour period. In contrast, most patients without glaucoma manifest a diurnal range of 2–6 mm Hg. Spontaneous fluctuations in IOP result in a diurnal pattern that is poorly reproducible, between days or between eyes. Also, in most healthy subjects and glaucoma patients, IOP has a distinct circadian rhythm, with peak pressures often occurring during sleep, particularly in the early-morning hours (see Chapter 2). About two-thirds of patients reach peak IOPs during nonoffice hours.

Thus, a single IOP measurement during office hours does not provide an accurate assessment of IOP variability over time. Table 4-1 lists some of the reasons that elevated IOP may be undetected in patients with high-tension glaucoma. Large diurnal fluctuation in IOP has been identified as an independent risk factor for progression of glaucoma in some

Table 4-1 Potential Reasons for Undetected High-Tension Glaucoma

Primary open-angle glaucoma with diurnal IOP fluctuation
Intermittent IOP elevation
   Nonacute angle-closure glaucoma
   Glaucomatocyclitic crisis
   Secondary glaucoma (eg, pigmentary, pseudoexfoliation, uveitic)
Normalized IOP in an eye with previously elevated IOP (eg, corticosteroid-induced, uveitic,
   pigmentary, hyphema)
Use of medications that may lower IOP (eg, systemic β-blocker)
Inaccurate IOP measurement (due to thin central cornea, reduced scleral rigidity, uncalibrated
   device, poor examiner technique)

IOP = intraocular pressure.

studies but not in others. Regardless, elevation of IOP is a strong risk factor for glaucoma progression.

As discussed in Chapter 2, central corneal thickness (CCT) affects the measurement of IOP. Thicker corneas resist the deformation inherent in most methods of tonometry, resulting in an overestimation of IOP. In contrast, tonometry in eyes with thin corneas underestimates the IOP. The average CCT in adult eyes, determined by ultrasonic pachymetry, ranges between 540 and 550 μm and varies with race and ethnicity. For example, in populations of persons of African ancestry, mean CCT is lower than in whites.

Bengtsson B, Leske MC, Hyman L, Heijl A; Early Manifest Glaucoma Trial Group. Fluctuation of intraocular pressure and glaucoma progression in the early manifest glaucoma trial. *Ophthalmology.* 2007;114(2):205–209.

Bhan A, Browning AC, Shah S, Hamilton R, Dave D, Dua HS. Effect of corneal thickness on intraocular pressure measurements with the pneumotonometer, Goldmann applanation tonometer, and Tono-Pen. *Invest Ophthalmol Vis Sci.* 2002;43(5):1389–1392.

Brandt JD, Beiser JA, Kass MA, Gordon MO. Central corneal thickness in the Ocular Hypertension Treatment Study (OHTS). *Ophthalmology.* 2001;108(10):1779–1788.

Doughty MJ, Zaman ML. Human corneal thickness and its impact on intraocular pressure measures: a review and meta-analysis approach. *Surv Ophthalmol.* 2000;44(5):367–408.

Liu JHK, Kripke DF, Twa MD, et al. Twenty-four-hour pattern of intraocular pressure in the aging population. *Invest Ophthalmol Vis Sci.* 1999;40(12):2912–2917.

Older age

The Baltimore Eye Survey found that the prevalence of glaucoma increases dramatically with age, particularly among individuals of African descent, whose prevalence exceeded 11% in those older than 80 years. In the Collaborative Initial Glaucoma Treatment Study (CIGTS; see Clinical Trial 4-1 at the end of this chapter), visual field defects were 7 times more likely to progress in patients 60 years or older than in those younger than 40 years. The Ocular Hypertension Treatment Study (OHTS; see Clinical Trial 4-2 at the end of this chapter) found an increased risk of progression to OAG with age (per decade): 43% in the univariate analysis and 22% in the multivariate analysis. In the general population, increased IOP is associated with increased age and may partially account for the observed relationship between age and glaucoma. However, studies from Japan have shown a relationship between increased age and glaucomatous progression in a population with sustained IOP. Therefore, older age appears to be an independent risk factor for the development and progression of glaucoma.

Race

The prevalence of POAG in the United States is 3–4 times greater in individuals of African descent or Hispanic ethnicity than in primarily European-derived populations. Blindness from glaucoma is at least 4 times more common in blacks than in whites. In addition, glaucoma is more likely to be diagnosed in black patients at a younger age and at a more advanced stage than it is in white patients. In the OHTS, glaucoma was 59% more likely to develop in black patients with ocular hypertension (defined in this study as elevated IOP in the absence of optic nerve or visual field abnormalities) than in white patients with ocular hypertension, in a univariate analysis. However, this relationship was not present after controlling for corneal thickness and baseline vertical cup–disc ratio in a multivariate analysis (black patients had overall thinner CCT and larger baseline vertical cup–disc ratios).

Thin central corneal thickness

A thinner cornea is an important risk factor for disease progression in individuals with POAG (with higher baseline IOPs) and for the development of glaucoma in individuals with ocular hypertension. This risk can be attributed, in part, to the underestimation of IOP measured by Goldmann tonometry in patients with thin corneas. In addition, thin corneas may be a biomarker for disease susceptibility. As mentioned previously, black patients have thinner corneas on average than white patients.

Positive family history

In the Baltimore Eye Survey, the relative risk of POAG increased approximately 3.7-fold for individuals who had a sibling with POAG.

Myopia

Population-based data support an association between POAG and myopia. In the Beaver Dam Eye Study, myopia (≤–1 D spherical equivalent) was significantly associated with a diagnosis of glaucoma. In the Rotterdam follow-up study, high myopia (≤–4 D spherical equivalent) was associated with an increased risk (2.31 times higher) of development of glaucoma. However, the OHTS did not find an association between myopia and the incidence of glaucoma.

The concurrence of POAG and myopia may complicate diagnosis and management in several ways. Evaluation of the optic nerve head is particularly challenging in highly myopic eyes that have tilted discs or posterior staphylomas. Also, the myopic refractive error may cause minification of the optic nerve, further complicating accurate optic nerve assessment. Myopia-related retinal degeneration or anomalies can cause visual field abnormalities that are difficult to distinguish from those caused by glaucoma. In addition, patients who are highly myopic may have difficulty performing accurately on visual field tests, making interpretation of visual field abnormalities more challenging.

Varma R, Ying-Lai M, Francis BA, et al; Los Angeles Latino Eye Study Group. Prevalence of open-angle glaucoma and ocular hypertension in Latinos: the Los Angeles Latino Eye Study. *Ophthalmology.* 2004;111(8):1439–1448.

Wilson MR, Martone JF. Epidemiology of chronic open-angle glaucoma. In: Ritch R, Shields MB, Krupin T. *The Glaucomas*. 2nd ed. St Louis: Mosby; 1996:753–768.

Wong TY, Klein BE, Klein R, Knudtson M, Lee KE. Refractive errors, intraocular pressure, and glaucoma in a white population. *Ophthalmology*. 2003;110(1):211–217.

Associated Disorders

Diabetes mellitus

There is controversy as to whether diabetes mellitus is a risk factor for glaucoma. The Beaver Dam Eye Study, the Blue Mountains Eye Study, and the Los Angeles Latino Eye Study found an association between diabetes and OAG. However, the Framingham Study, the Baltimore Eye Survey, the Barbados Eye Study, and a revised analysis of the Rotter- dam Study did not find a significant association. Furthermore, the Rotterdam Study and the Barbados Eye Study, which were large longitudinal population-based studies, did not identify diabetes as a risk factor for the development of glaucoma. In the OHTS, diabetes was associated with a reduced risk of developing glaucoma. However, the cohort of dia- betic patients was skewed, because the presence of retinopathy was an exclusion criterion for this study.

de Voogd S, Ikram MK, Wolfs RC, et al. Is diabetes mellitus a risk factor for open-angle glaucoma? The Rotterdam Study. *Ophthalmology*. 2006;113(10):1827–1831.

Hypertension

The Baltimore Eye Survey found that systemic hypertension was associated with a lower risk of glaucoma in younger (<65 years) subjects and a higher risk of glaucoma in older subjects. The hypothesis is that younger individuals with high blood pressure may have better perfusion of the optic nerve, but as these patients age, their chronic hypertension may have adverse effects on the microcirculation of the optic nerve and increase its sus- ceptibility to glaucomatous optic neuropathy. Conversely, in the Barbados Eye Study, the relative risk of developing glaucoma among subjects with systemic hypertension was less than 1.0 in all age groups, including those aged 70 years and older.

Lower ocular perfusion pressure

There is compelling evidence that lower ocular perfusion pressure (OPP; often defined as diastolic blood pressure + 1/3 systolic blood pressure – IOP) is a risk factor for the devel- opment of glaucoma. Although this definition of OPP oversimplifies actual ocular blood flow, several factors, including autoregulatory mechanisms in central nervous system perfusion, make the association between OPP and glaucoma intriguing. The overtreat- ment of systemic hypertension may contribute to glaucoma progression in some cases (eg, normal-tension glaucoma) and should be monitored. Clinicians should consider measuring a patient's blood pressure in the office, particularly if the patient is starting a β-adrenergic blocking medication.

Leske MC, Wu SY, Hennis A, Honkanen R, Nemesure B; BESs Study Group. Risk factors for incident open-angle glaucoma: the Barbados Eye Studies. *Ophthalmology*. 2008;115(1): 85–93.

Retinal vein occlusion

In patients with central retinal vein occlusion (CRVO), elevated IOP due to neovascularization of the angle may progress to glaucoma. Thus, routine gonioscopy should be performed in these patients. Also, susceptible individuals with elevated IOP (ie, ocular hypertension or glaucoma) are at risk of developing CRVO. Consideration should be given to treating elevated IOP in patients with a history of CRVO in order to reduce the risk of CRVO in the fellow eye. As the pathophysiology of hemicentral retinal vein occlusion is similar to that of CRVO, treatment considerations should be similar.

Other associated conditions

Sleep apnea, thyroid disorders, hypercholesterolemia, migraine headaches, low cerebrospinal fluid pressure, corneal hysteresis, and Raynaud phenomenon have variously been identified in some studies as potential risk factors for the development of glaucoma. Further research is required in order to clarify the significance of these conditions in patients with POAG and their relationship to glaucoma, if any.

Prognosis and Therapy

Most patients with POAG retain useful vision for their entire lives. The patients at greatest risk of blindness are those who present with visual field loss at the time of diagnosis. In a recent study, the cumulative risk of unilateral and bilateral blindness in patients with OAG was 7.4% and 3.4%, respectively, within 10 years of diagnosis, and 13.5% and 4.3%, respectively, within 20 years of diagnosis.

Treatment with topical medication, laser surgery, and incisional surgery to lower IOP has been shown to significantly reduce the risk of glaucomatous progression (see Clinical Trials 4-1 through 4-4 at the end of this chapter). For patients with decreased visual function, a referral to a vision rehabilitation specialist should be considered. These specialists can help improve visual function by optimizing lighting, enhancing contrast, reducing glare, and providing adaptations to enhance activities of daily living. Orientation and mobility specialists can be consulted and vision substitution strategies (eg, talking books, watches) utilized to improve daily function and quality of life for these patients. Additional information on vision rehabilitation, including patient handouts, is available on the American Academy of Ophthalmology website at https://www.aao.org/low-vision-and-vision-rehab. See BCSC Section 3, *Clinical Optics,* for in-depth discussion of low vision aids.

American Academy of Ophthalmology Glaucoma Panel. Preferred Practice Pattern Guidelines. *Primary Open-Angle Glaucoma.* San Francisco: American Academy of Ophthalmology; 2010. Available at www.aao.org/ppp.

American Academy of Ophthalmology Vision Rehabilitation Committee. Preferred Practice Pattern Guidelines. *Vision Rehabilitation.* San Francisco: American Academy of Ophthalmology; 2013. Available at www.aao.org/ppp.

Grover DS, Smith O. Recent clinical pearls from clinical trials in glaucoma. *Curr Opin Ophthalmol.* 2012;23(2):127–134.

Malihi M, Moura Filho ER, Hodge DO, Sit AJ. Long-term trends in glaucoma-related blindness in Olmsted County, Minnesota. *Ophthalmology.* 2014;121(1):134–141.

Open-Angle Glaucoma Without Elevated IOP (Normal-Tension Glaucoma, Low-Tension Glaucoma)

Controversy remains as to whether normal-tension glaucoma (NTG) represents a distinct disease entity or whether it is simply POAG developing with IOP within the statistically normal range. Glaucoma can develop at any level of IOP within the range observed in the general population. Thus, IOP is a continuous risk factor for glaucoma, and any cutoff between "normal" and "abnormal" IOP is arbitrary. Accordingly, many authorities believe the terms *normal-tension glaucoma* and *low-tension glaucoma* should be abandoned.

Risk Factors and Clinical Features

As previously emphasized, glaucoma is a multifactorial disease process for which elevated IOP is just one of several risk factors. Studies suggest that among persons of Japanese descent, the proportion of OAG with IOPs in the average range is particularly high. Other risk factors may play a greater role in NTG than in POAG with higher IOPs (ie, high-tension POAG). Many authorities hypothesize that local vascular factors may have a significant role in the development of NTG. Some studies suggest that patients with NTG have a higher prevalence of vasospastic disorders (eg, migraine and Raynaud phenomenon), ischemic vascular disease, autoimmune disease, sleep apnea, systemic hypotension, and coagulopathies than patients with high-tension POAG. However, these findings have not been consistent. Vascular autoregulatory defects have also been described in eyes with NTG.

NTG is characteristically bilateral but often asymmetric. In glaucomatous eyes with IOPs within the statistically normal range but asymmetric, worse damage typically occurs in the eye with the higher IOP. Optic disc hemorrhage (Fig 4-1) may be more common

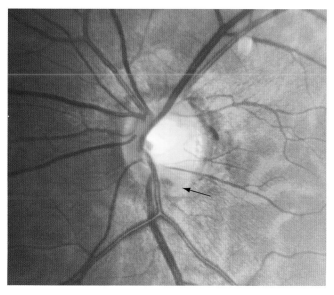

Figure 4-1 Subtle disc hemorrhage *(arrow)* in a patient with normal-tension glaucoma. *(Courtesy of Wallace L. M. Alward, MD. © The University of Iowa.)*

among patients with NTG than with high-tension POAG. Some authorities classify NTG into 2 groups based on optic nerve appearance:

- a *senile sclerotic group* with shallow, pale sloping of the neuroretinal rim that is primarily seen in older patients with vascular disease
- a *focal ischemic group* with deep, focal notching of the neuroretinal rim

The visual field defects in NTG tend to be more focal, deeper, and closer to fixation, especially with early disease, compared with those commonly seen with high-tension POAG. Also, a dense paracentral scotoma encroaching near fixation (ie, "shotgun" appearance) is not an unusual initial finding on the visual field tests of NTG patients. However, these differences may be due to detection bias. Further, differences in optic nerve appearance and visual field defects between patients with NTG and those with high-tension POAG are not uniformly confirmed in studies. Therefore, for any individual patient, there is no characteristic abnormality of the optic nerve or visual field that distinguishes NTG from high-tension POAG.

Cartwright MJ, Anderson DR. Correlation of asymmetric damage with asymmetric intraocular pressure in normal-tension glaucoma (low-tension glaucoma). *Arch Ophthalmol.*
1988;106(7):898–900.

Collaborative Normal-Tension Glaucoma Study Group. Comparison of glaucomatous
progression between untreated patients with normal-tension glaucoma and patients
with therapeutically reduced intraocular pressures. *Am J Ophthalmol.* 1998;126(4):
487–497.

Differential Diagnosis

Normal-tension glaucoma can be mimicked by many conditions, as summarized in Table 4-2. It is essential to distinguish NTG and other glaucomas from nonglaucomatous etiologies (eg, optic nerve drusen, ischemic optic neuropathy), because appropriate therapy may vary greatly. Visual field defects in several of these conditions may appear similar to those seen with NTG and can even be progressive.

POAG may be misdiagnosed as NTG because of diurnal variations of IOP. Diurnal IOP measurement may help determine target IOPs by identifying peak IOPs and IOP fluctuation, but it does not capture nocturnal patterns of IOP. Also, elevated IOP can be obscured in patients taking systemic medication, particularly systemic β-blockers. In addition, some patients with apparent NTG may have artifactually low tonometry readings because of reduced scleral rigidity or thin CCT. Similarly, decreased corneal thickness in

---

Table 4-2 Differential Diagnosis for Glaucomatous Optic Neuropathy

Congenital anomalies (eg, coloboma, optic nerve pit, myopic optic discs)
Physiologic cupping due to a large scleral canal
Optic nerve drusen
Compressive lesions of the optic nerve and chiasm
Anterior ischemic optic neuropathy
Posterior ischemic optic neuropathy
Toxic or nutritional optic neuropathy (eg, methanol, vitamin B_{12} deficiency)

---

patients who have undergone refractive surgery may result in an erroneous diagnosis of NTG because of an underestimation of true IOP. Patients with myopia may have anomalous optic nerve heads or myopia-related visual field defects that often make it difficult to diagnose glaucoma or monitor for glaucomatous progression.

Diagnostic Evaluation

The clinician must carefully review the patient's medical history for conditions that cause an optic nerve appearance and/or visual field defects similar to those seen in NTG: these include significant systemic hemorrhage associated with low blood pressure, myocardial infarction, or shock. Visual field defects consistent with glaucoma have been noted after a decrease in blood pressure following a hypotensive crisis; however, these defects do not progress once the underlying condition is stable. It is also important to inquire about previous corticosteroid use associated with prior glaucomatous damage that has stabilized. Further, obtaining a detailed medical history is important to assess for conditions associated with NTG, such as migraine headaches, autoimmune disease, sleep apnea, and chronic or nocturnal low blood pressure.

Before confirming a diagnosis of NTG, the clinician should measure the patient's IOP by applanation tonometry at various times of the day (ie, diurnal curve), as well as on different days. Repeated testing may detect elevated IOP in many of these eyes. Gonioscopy should be performed to rule out other etiologies, such as angle closure, trauma (ie, angle recession), prior inflammation, or pigment dispersion. Careful stereoscopic optic nerve evaluation is essential to rule out other congenital or acquired optic nerve anomalies, such as a coloboma, drusen, or physiologic cupping due to a large scleral canal.

In the setting of atypical findings—for example, unilateral disease, decreased central vision, dyschromatopsia, young age, presence of a relative afferent pupillary defect, neuroretinal rim pallor, or visual field loss inconsistent with optic nerve appearance—additional medical and neurologic evaluation should be considered. This may include evaluation for anemia, carotid artery insufficiency, syphilis, certain vitamin deficiencies, temporal arteritis, or other causes of systemic vasculitis. Auscultation and palpation of the carotid arteries should be performed; noninvasive tests of carotid circulation (eg, carotid Doppler ultrasonography) may be helpful. In cases of optic nerve pallor or visual field loss suggestive of a neurologic defect, evaluation of the optic nerve and chiasm with computed tomography or magnetic resonance imaging may be warranted. See also BCSC Section 5, *Neuro-Ophthalmology.*

Greenfield DS, Siatkowski RM, Glaser JS, Schatz NJ, Parrish RK II. The cupped disc. Who needs neuroimaging? *Ophthalmology.* 1998;105(10):1866–1874.

Prognosis and Therapy

In the Collaborative Normal-Tension Glaucoma Study (CNTGS), IOP lowering by at least 30% reduced the 5-year risk of visual field progression from 35% to 12%, supporting the role of IOP in NTG. It should be noted that the protective effect of IOP reduction was evident only after adjusting for the effect of cataracts, which were more frequent in the treated group. Based on the findings of the CNTGS, treatment of NTG is generally recommended unless the optic neuropathy is determined to be stable. Interestingly, 65% of patients in this study did not progress over the study duration despite no treatment, whereas 12% of patients progressed despite a 30% reduction of IOP. Factors in addition to IOP are likely operative in patients with this disease. The rate of visual field progression was highly variable yet slow in most individuals with visual field progression. In addition, this study showed a lower treatment benefit among patients with a baseline history of a disc hemorrhage.

The initial goal of therapy is often to achieve a near 30% IOP reduction from a carefully determined baseline IOP. Once this is established, routine evaluations with appropriate individualized adjustments for target pressure are recommended. These adjustments should take into account relevant factors, including baseline severity of optic nerve damage and visual field loss, potential risks of therapy, comorbid conditions, and life expectancy of the patient. Target pressure should be reassessed and adjusted as needed during follow-up visits in order to maintain visual function.

To achieve the target IOP, medications, laser trabeculoplasty, or filtering surgery may be indicated. Topical medical therapy is the most common initial approach in the management of NTG. In addition to lowering IOP, some glaucoma medications may have neuroprotective properties or may improve ocular perfusion. These potential benefits have not been proven clinically, and the role of neuroprotective agents remains under investigation. Some glaucoma specialists are wary of treating NTG with topical β-blocker medications because of their association with low ocular perfusion pressure (see the subsection "Lower ocular perfusion pressure"). The Low-Pressure Glaucoma Treatment Study (LoGTS) showed a high rate of glaucomatous progression in patients treated with timolol. However, there was a significant loss of follow-up in this study; the results must be interpreted with caution. In the Early Manifest Glaucoma Trial (EMGT; see Clinical Trial 4-3), IOP-lowering with the combination of betaxolol and argon laser trabeculoplasty (ALT) was minimal in eyes with baseline IOPs of 15 mm Hg or lower. This suggests that patients with a lower baseline IOP who are progressing may need incisional surgery or medications other than β-blockers to stabilize their disease. See Chapter 8 for further discussion of indications for surgery. The use of an adjunct antifibrotic agent (eg, mitomycin C or 5-fluorouracil) during filtering surgery may improve the likelihood that the target IOP will be reached.

Bhandari A, Crabb DP, Poinoosawmy D, Fitzke FW, Hitchings RA, Noureddin BN. Effect of surgery on visual field progression in normal-tension glaucoma. *Ophthalmology.* 1997;104(7):1131–1137.

Collaborative Normal-Tension Glaucoma Study Group. Comparison of glaucomatous progression between untreated patients with normal-tension glaucoma and patients with therapeutically reduced intraocular pressures. *Am J Ophthalmol.* 1998;126(4): 487–497.

Collaborative Normal-Tension Glaucoma Study Group. The effectiveness of intraocular pressure reduction in the treatment of normal-tension glaucoma. *Am J Ophthalmol.* 1998; 126(4):498–505.

Mikelberg FS. Normal tension glaucoma. *Focal Points: Clinical Modules for Ophthalmologists.* San Francisco: American Academy of Ophthalmology; 2000, module 12.

The Glaucoma Suspect

A glaucoma suspect is defined as an individual who has either (1) a suspicious optic nerve or nerve fiber layer appearance in the absence of a visual field defect; or (2) a visual field defect suggestive of glaucoma in the absence of a corresponding glaucomatous optic nerve abnormality. Patients with such findings are typically monitored for the development of glaucoma with periodic evaluation of the optic nerve, retinal nerve fiber layer, and visual field. In patients with an absence of visual field defects on standard perimetry (see Chapter 3), the use of frequency-doubling technology and pattern electroretinogram may be useful for detecting early loss of visual function. If signs of optic nerve damage are present, the diagnosis of early POAG and initiation of treatment should be considered. In uncertain cases, however, close monitoring of the patient without treatment is reasonable in order to better establish a diagnosis (ie, confirm initial findings or detect progressive changes) before initiation of therapy. Glaucoma suspects who have elevated IOP and structural or functional findings that are not firmly diagnostic of glaucoma may be difficult to classify into one diagnostic category.

Ocular Hypertension

Some authors consider patients with ocular hypertension to be glaucoma suspects. In this book, *ocular hypertension* is defined as a condition in which IOP is elevated above an arbitrary cutoff value, typically 21 mm Hg, in the absence of optic nerve, retinal nerve fiber layer, or visual field abnormalities. Estimates of the prevalence of ocular hypertension in the United States vary considerably and may be as high as 8 times that of diagnosed POAG. Studies of individuals with elevated IOP for various lengths of time suggest that a higher baseline IOP is associated with a greater risk of developing glaucoma. However, for most persons with elevated IOP, the risk of developing glaucoma is low.

Distinguishing between ocular hypertension and early POAG is often difficult. The ophthalmologist must look carefully for signs of early damage to the optic nerve, such as focal notching, asymmetry of cupping, optic disc hemorrhage, nerve fiber layer defects, or subtle visual field defects.

There is no clear consensus about whether elevated IOP should be treated in the absence of signs of early damage. Some clinicians, after assessing all risk factors, select and treat those individuals thought to be at greatest risk of developing glaucoma. In the OHTS, patients 40–80 years of age with IOP between 24 and 32 mm Hg were randomized to either observation or treatment with topical ocular hypotensive medications (see Clinical Trial 4-2 at the end of this chapter). During a 5-year period, 4.4% of participants in the treatment group versus 9.5% of participants in the observation group progressed to glaucoma, based on optic nerve and visual field changes. Thus, topical medications reduce the risk of progression to glaucoma in patients with ocular hypertension. It should be noted, however, that most untreated participants did not progress over a 5-year period. In the OHTS, the risk of developing glaucoma was increased by 10% for every mm Hg increase in IOP from the baseline IOP; the risk was increased by 32% for each 0.1 increment in vertical cup–disc ratio.

Results from the OHTS suggest that increased age, higher IOP, thinner corneas, larger cup–disc ratio at baseline, and higher pattern standard deviation on standard automated perimetry are important risk factors for the development of POAG. Data from the OHTS and the European Glaucoma Prevention Study were combined to create a risk calculation model to predict the 5-year risk of conversion from ocular hypertension to glaucoma based on these risk factors. The increased risk of glaucoma progression attributed to thinner corneas in the OHTS, however, was not fully explained by the estimated artifactual error in measured IOP. This may be due to thinner corneas being a biomarker for other susceptibility factors. The increased risk of glaucoma progression in black participants (on univariate but not multivariate analyses) may be attributed to their thinner corneas and greater cup–disc ratios. Interestingly, a positive family history of glaucoma was not identified as a significant risk factor in this study, possibly because of inadequate assessment from self-reporting. Clinicians should consider family history when evaluating a patient's risk of glaucoma. Other potential risk factors, such as myopia, diabetes mellitus, migraine, and high or low blood pressure, were not confirmed in the OHTS as significant risk factors for glaucomatous progression.

Initial reports from the OHTS clearly demonstrate that lowering IOP in individuals with ocular hypertension reduces the risk of progression to glaucoma. It is important to recognize, however, that the incremental structural or functional change that constituted a progression endpoint in the OHTS would likely not manifest as symptomatic vision loss. Therefore, the question remains whether delaying treatment is associated with poorer outcomes compared with early initiation of IOP-lowering therapy. The results from the OHTS suggest that clinicians may safely consider delaying the treatment of ocular hypertension, particularly among patients with a lower risk of conversion to glaucoma (see Clinical Trial 4-2 at the end of this chapter).

The decision of whether to treat a patient with ocular hypertension should be based on results from the OHTS, findings from the clinical examination, and discussions with the patient. The clinician and patient should consider whether the risk factors for developing glaucoma outweigh the inconvenience, cost, and potential side effects of therapy for the patient. Additional factors to consider include the patient's age, potential life span, adherence to therapy and follow-up visits, and the ability to monitor disease progression with accurate assessments of the optic nerve (eg, anomalous optic nerves may be difficult to monitor) and reliable visual field tests.

American Academy of Ophthalmology Glaucoma Panel. Preferred Practice Pattern Guidelines. *Primary Open-Angle Glaucoma Suspect.* San Francisco: American Academy of Ophthalmology; 2010. Available at www.aao.org/ppp.

Gordon MO, Beiser JA, Brandt JD, et al. The Ocular Hypertension Treatment Study: baseline factors that predict the onset of primary open-angle glaucoma. *Arch Ophthalmol.* 2002; 120(6):714–720.

Kass MA, Gordon MO, Gao F, et al. Delaying treatment of ocular hypertension: the ocular hypertension treatment study. *Arch Ophthalmol.* 2010;128(3):276–287.

Kass MA, Heuer DK, Higginbotham EJ, et al. The Ocular Hypertension Treatment Study: a randomized trial determines that topical ocular hypotensive medication delays or prevents the onset of primary open-angle glaucoma. *Arch Ophthalmol.* 2002;120(6):701–713.

Wilson MR, Brandt JD. Update on glaucoma clinical trials. *Focal Points: Clinical Modules for Ophthalmologists.* American Academy of Ophthalmology; 2003, module 9.

Secondary Open-Angle Glaucoma

Pseudoexfoliation Syndrome

Pseudoexfoliation syndrome (exfoliation syndrome) is characterized by the deposition of a distinctive fibrillar extracellular material in the anterior segment of the eye. Histologically, this material has been found in and on the lens epithelium and capsule, pupillary margin, ciliary epithelium, iris pigment epithelium, iris stroma, iris blood vessels, and subconjunctival tissue. The material has also been identified in other parts of the body. Mutations in a single gene, *LOXL1,* seem to be present in nearly all cases of pseudoexfoliation syndrome and pseudoexfoliation glaucoma; however, these disease-associated mutations are also common in populations without pseudoexfoliation syndrome or glaucoma, suggesting a multifactorial etiology for this disease. The exact mechanism by which *LOXL1* mutations are related to pseudoexfoliation syndrome is unclear, but it likely involves the reduced or abnormal synthesis of elastin fibers. Pseudoexfoliation syndrome may be a systemic disease with material deposits found in various organs, including the skin, lung, heart, and liver.

Pseudoexfoliation syndrome can present unilaterally or bilaterally and with varying degrees of asymmetry. Often, this disorder presents unilaterally, and the uninvolved eye manifests signs of the disease at a later time. This syndrome is strongly age related: it is rarely seen in persons younger than 50 years and occurs most commonly in individuals older than 70 years.

The classic characteristic of pseudoexfoliation syndrome is the deposition of fibrillar deposits in a "bull's-eye" pattern on the anterior lens capsule, which is best seen after pupillary dilation. This pattern is presumably caused by iris movement that scrapes the pseudoexfoliative material from the lens, causing a clear intermediate area in between a central and peripheral zone of the material (Fig 4-2). Clinically, this fibrillar extracellular material

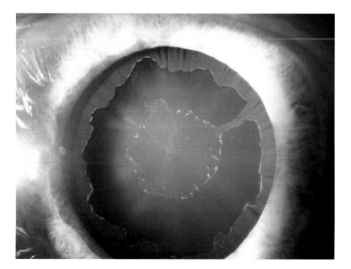

Figure 4-2 Pseudoexfoliation syndrome. Pseudoexfoliative material deposited on the anterior lens capsule in a classic bull's-eye pattern in a dilated eye. *(Courtesy of Wallace L. M. Alward, MD. From the Iowa Glaucoma Curriculum [curriculum.iowaglaucoma.org]. © The University of Iowa.)*

can be seen on the pupillary margin, zonular fibers of the lens, ciliary processes, inferior anterior chamber angle, corneal endothelium, and the anterior hyaloid (Figs 4-3, 4-4).

Individuals with pseudoexfoliation syndrome may also have peripupillary atrophy with transillumination defects. These patients may have fine pigment deposits on the iris or in a vertical linear pattern on the cornea (Krukenberg spindles); the deposits are also commonly seen in persons with pigmentary dispersion syndrome. The pupil often dilates poorly, likely because of infiltration of fibrillar material into the iris stroma. Phacodonesis and iridodonesis can be seen and are due to the weak zonular fibers. Thus, great care must be taken during cataract surgery to reduce the risk of zonular dehiscence, vitreous loss,

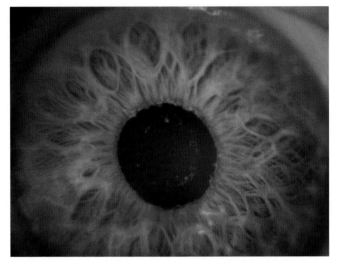

Figure 4-3 Pseudoexfoliative material deposited on the pupillary margin and anterior lens capsule in an undilated eye. *(Courtesy of Wallace L. M. Alward, MD. From the* Iowa Glaucoma Curriculum *[curriculum .iowaglaucoma.org]. © The University of Iowa.)*

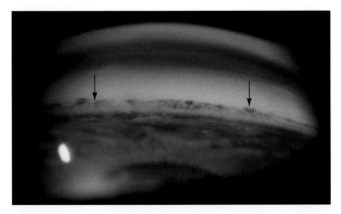

Figure 4-4 Goniophotograph of pseudoexfoliative debris deposited in the anterior chamber angle. Note the Sampaolesi line *(arrows)*. *(Courtesy of Wallace L. M. Alward, MD. From the* Iowa Glaucoma Curriculum *[curriculum.iowaglaucoma.org]. © The University of Iowa.)*

lens dislocation, and other complications intraoperatively and postoperatively (see also BCSC Section 11, *Lens and Cataract*). Iris angiography has shown abnormalities of the iris vessels with leakage of fluorescein.

On gonioscopy, the trabecular meshwork is typically heavily pigmented, sometimes in a variegated fashion. Pigment deposition anterior to the Schwalbe line is commonly seen and referred to as the *Sampaolesi line* (see Fig 4-4). The zonular fibers in patients with pseudoexfoliation syndrome are often weak and may cause an anterior movement of the lens–iris interface, resulting in narrow angles.

The IOP elevation associated with pseudoexfoliation syndrome is likely due to deposits of fibrillar material in the trabecular meshwork that impede the outflow of aqueous through the trabecular meshwork or uveoscleral pathways. In addition, since elastin is an important component of the lamina cribrosa, pseudoexfoliation syndrome may increase the susceptibility of the optic nerve to injury. This increased susceptibility may, in turn, contribute to the increased risk of development and progression of glaucoma in these patients, as was found in the Early Manifest Glaucoma Trial (see Clinical Trial 4-3 at the end of this chapter).

Individuals with pseudoexfoliation syndrome with elevated IOP resulting in optic nerve damage or visual field loss are described as having *pseudoexfoliation glaucoma*. Pseudoexfoliation syndrome is associated with OAG in all populations, but the prevalence varies considerably. In Scandinavian countries, pseudoexfoliation syndrome accounts for more than 50% of cases of OAG. The risk of progression to glaucoma also varies widely and can be as high as 40% of patients over a 10-year period. Pseudoexfoliation glaucoma differs from POAG in that it often presents unilaterally and with greater pigmentation of the trabecular meshwork. In addition, the IOP is often higher and there are greater diurnal fluctuations in IOP in pseudoexfoliation glaucoma than in POAG. The overall prognosis for glaucoma is worse for patients with pseudoexfoliation glaucoma than for those with POAG. Laser trabeculoplasty can be very effective, but the duration of the response may be shorter in pseudoexfoliation glaucoma than in POAG. Lens extraction does not alleviate the condition.

Anastasopoulos E, Founti P, Topouzis F. Update on pseudoexfoliation syndrome pathogenesis and associations with intraocular pressure, glaucoma and systemic diseases. *Curr Opin Ophthalmol.* 2015;26(2):82–89.

Thorleifsson G, Magnusson KP, Sulem P, et al. Common sequence variants in the *LOXL1* gene confer susceptibility to exfoliation glaucoma. *Science.* 2007;317(5843):1397–1400.

Pigment Dispersion Syndrome

In pigment dispersion syndrome, the zonular fibers rub the posterior iris pigment epithelium, resulting in the release of pigment granules throughout the eye. Posterior bowing of the iris with "reverse pupillary block" configuration is noted in many eyes with pigment dispersion syndrome. This concave iris configuration results in greater contact with the zonular fibers, causing increased release of pigment granules.

Pigment dispersion syndrome classically presents with pigment deposits on the corneal endothelium, trabecular meshwork, and lens periphery, as well as with midperipheral iris transillumination defects in a spokelike pattern. The pigment deposits on the corneal endothelium are typically in a vertical spindle pattern, referred to as *Krukenberg spindle* (Fig 4-5), and are caused by aqueous convection currents and subsequent phago-cytosis of pigment by the corneal endothelium. The presence of a Krukenberg spindle is not necessary for a diagnosis of pigment dispersion syndrome, however, and this sign may be present in other diseases, such as pseudoexfoliation syndrome. The midperiph-eral iris transillumination defects are a result of contact between the zonular fibers and the posterior iris pigment epithelium (Fig 4-6). On gonioscopy, the trabecular meshwork commonly appears as homogeneous and densely pigmented, with speckled pigment at or anterior to the Schwalbe line (Fig 4-7), often forming a Sampaolesi line. When the eye is dilated, pigment deposits may be seen on the zonular fibers, on the anterior hya-loid, and in the equatorial region of the lens capsule (Zentmayer ring or Scheie stripe, Fig 4-8).

With increasing age, the signs of pigment dispersion may decrease as a result of nor-mal growth of the lens, inducing a physiologic pupillary block and anterior movement of the iris. Loss of accommodation may also occur. As pigment dispersion is reduced,

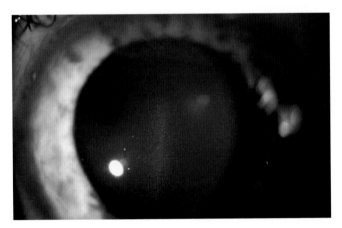

Figure 4-5 Krukenberg spindle in a patient with pigmentary glaucoma. *(Reproduced from Alward WLM, Longmuir RA. Color Atlas of Gonioscopy. 2nd ed. San Francisco: American Academy of Ophthalmology; 2008:75. Fig 9-1.)*

Figure 4-6 Goniophotograph of the classic spokelike iris transillumination defects of pig-ment dispersion syndrome. *(Courtesy of Angelo P. Tanna, MD.)*

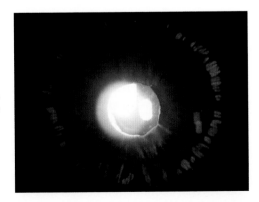

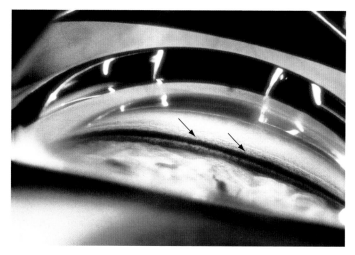

Figure 4-7 Characteristic heavy, uniform pigmentation of the trabecular meshwork *(arrows)* occurring in pigment dispersion syndrome and pigmentary glaucoma. *(Courtesy of M. Roy Wilson, MD.)*

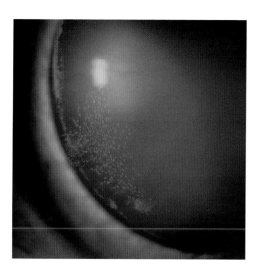

Figure 4-8 In pigment dispersion syndrome, pigment deposits are visible in the equatorial region of the lens capsule (Zentmayer ring or Scheie stripe) and on the zonular fibers. *(Courtesy of Angelo P. Tanna, MD.)*

the deposited pigment may fade from the corneal endothelium, trabecular meshwork, or anterior surface of the iris.

Approximately 15% of individuals with pigment dispersion syndrome progress to glaucoma or elevated IOP requiring treatment. Pigmentary glaucoma is 3 times more common in men than in women, particularly men who are young or middle-aged (20–50 years) and myopic. The presumed mechanism of elevated IOP is obstruction of the trabecular meshwork by pigment granules. *Pigmentary glaucoma* is characterized by wide fluctuations in IOP, which can exceed 50 mm Hg in untreated eyes. Affected patients may have extreme elevations in IOP following exercise or pupillary dilation because of an excessive liberation of pigment. Symptoms associated with such elevated IOPs may include halos, intermittent blurry vision, and ocular pain.

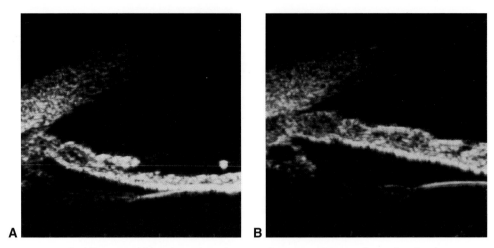

Figure 4-9 **A,** Ultrasound biomicroscopy image of concave iris configuration in pigmentary glaucoma, before laser peripheral iridotomy (LPI). **B,** Same eye, after LPI. *(Courtesy of Charles J. Pavlin, MD.)*

Laser peripheral iridotomy has been proposed as a means of minimizing posterior bowing of the iris (Fig 4-9). However, its effectiveness in treating pigmentary glaucoma has not been established. Medical treatment is often successful in reducing elevated IOP. Patients respond reasonably well to laser trabeculoplasty, although the effect may be short-lived. Because the heavy trabecular meshwork pigmentation allows increased absorption of laser energy, lower-energy settings are recommended during laser trabeculoplasty to avoid an acute rise in IOP after treatment. Filtering surgery is usually successful; however, extra care is warranted in young myopic male patients, who are at increased risk for hypotony maculopathy.

Niyadurupola N, Broadway DC. Pigment dispersion syndrome and pigmentary glaucoma— a major review. *Clin Experiment Ophthalmol.* 2008;36(9):868–882.

Reistad CE, Shields MB, Campbell DG, et al; American Glaucoma Society Pigmentary Glaucoma Iridotomy Study Group. The influence of peripheral iridotomy on the intraocular pressure course in patients with pigmentary glaucoma. *J Glaucoma.* 2005;14(4):255–259.

Siddiqui Y, Ten Hulzen RD, Cameron JD, Hodge DO, Johnson DH. What is the risk of developing pigmentary glaucoma from pigment dispersion syndrome? *Am J Ophthalmol.* 2003;135(6):794–799.

Lens-Induced Glaucoma

The lens can play a causative role in the development of open-angle and angle-closure glaucoma. Lens-induced OAGs are divided into 3 clinical entities:

- phacolytic glaucoma
- lens particle glaucoma
- phacoantigenic glaucoma

Lens-induced angle-closure glaucomas include phacomorphic glaucoma and ectopia lentis and are discussed in Chapter 5. See also BCSC Section 9, *Uveitis and Ocular Inflammation,* and Section 11, *Lens and Cataract.*

Phacolytic glaucoma

Phacolytic glaucoma is an inflammatory glaucoma caused by the leakage of high-molecular-weight lens protein through the capsule of a mature or hypermature cataract (Fig 4-10) that subsequently obstructs the trabecular meshwork. As the lens ages, its protein composition becomes altered, with an increased concentration of high-molecular-weight lens protein. In a mature or hypermature cataract, these proteins are released through microscopic openings in the lens capsule. Elevated IOP occurs as a result of obstruction of the trabecular meshwork by these high-molecular-weight proteins, lens-laden macrophages, and other inflammatory debris.

Individuals with phacolytic glaucoma are usually older patients with a history of poor vision. They have a sudden onset of pain, conjunctival hyperemia, and worsening vision. Examination reveals markedly elevated IOP, microcystic corneal edema, prominent cell and flare reaction without keratic precipitates (KP), an open anterior chamber angle, and a mature or hypermature cataract (Fig 4-11). The lack of KPs helps distinguish phacolytic glaucoma from phacoantigenic glaucoma. Cellular debris may be seen layered in the anterior chamber angle, and a pseudohypopyon may be present. Large white particles (clumps of lens protein) may also be seen in the anterior chamber. The mature or hypermature

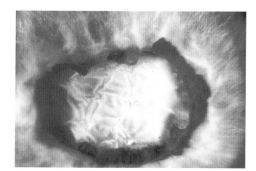

Figure 4-10 Characteristic appearance of hypermature cataract with wrinkling of the anterior lens capsule, which results from loss of cortical volume. Extensive posterior synechiae are present, which suggests previous inflammation. *(Courtesy of Steven T. Simmons, MD.)*

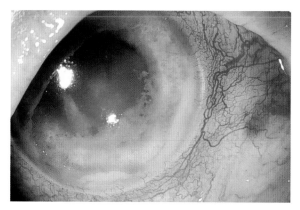

Figure 4-11 Phacolytic glaucoma. The typical presentation of phacolytic glaucoma is conjunctival hyperemia, microcystic corneal edema, mature cataract, and prominent anterior chamber reaction, as demonstrated in this photograph. Note the lens protein deposits on the endothelium and layering in the angle, creating a pseudohypopyon. *(Courtesy of George A. Cioffi, MD.)*

(morgagnian) cataract may have wrinkling of the anterior lens capsule, which represents loss of volume and the release of lens material (see Fig 4-10). Ocular hypotensive medications to reduce the IOP should be used immediately; however, definitive therapy requires cataract extraction.

Lens particle glaucoma

In lens particle glaucoma, retention of lens material in the eye after cataract extraction, capsulotomy, or ocular trauma results in obstruction of the trabecular meshwork. The severity of IOP elevation depends on the quantity of lens material released, the degree of inflammation, the ability of the trabecular meshwork to clear the lens material, and the functional status of the ciliary body, which is often altered following surgery or trauma.

Lens particle glaucoma usually occurs within weeks of the initial surgery or trauma, but it may occur months or years later. Clinical findings include cortical material in the anterior chamber, elevated IOP, moderate anterior chamber reaction, microcystic corneal edema, and, with time, posterior synechiae and peripheral anterior synechiae (PAS).

Medical therapy should be initiated to reduce the IOP while the residual lens material resorbs. Appropriate therapy includes medications to decrease aqueous formation, mydriatics to inhibit posterior synechiae formation, and topical corticosteroids to reduce inflammation. If the IOP cannot be controlled, surgical removal of the lens material is necessary.

Phacoantigenic glaucoma

Phacoantigenic glaucoma (previously known as *phacoanaphylaxis*) is a rare entity in which patients become sensitized to their own lens protein following surgery or penetrating trauma, resulting in a granulomatous inflammation. The clinical picture is quite varied, but most patients present with a moderate anterior chamber reaction with KPs on both the corneal endothelium and the anterior lens surface. In addition, a low-grade vitritis, posterior synechiae and PAS, and residual lens material in the anterior chamber may be present. Glaucomatous optic neuropathy may occur, but it is not common in eyes with phacoantigenic glaucoma. Initiation of topical corticosteroids and aqueous suppressants are recommended to reduce the inflammation and IOP. If medical treatment is unsuccessful, residual lens material should be removed.

Intraocular Tumors

A variety of tumors can cause unilateral chronic glaucoma. Many of the tumors described in this section are also discussed in BCSC Section 4, *Ophthalmic Pathology and Intraocular Tumors*. Glaucoma can result from several different mechanisms, depending on the size, type, and location of the tumor:

- direct tumor invasion of the anterior chamber angle
- angle closure by rotation of the ciliary body or by anterior displacement of the lens–iris interface (see Chapter 5)
- intraocular hemorrhage
- neovascularization of the angle
- deposition of tumor cells, inflammatory cells, and cellular debris within the trabecular meshwork

Choroidal and retinal tumors typically cause a secondary angle-closure glaucoma by the anterior displacement of the lens–iris diaphragm, resulting in closure of the anterior chamber angle. Posterior synechiae may develop as a result of inflammation of necrotic tumors; they exacerbate angle closure through a pupillary block mechanism. Choroidal melanomas, medulloepitheliomas, and retinoblastomas may also cause neovascularization of the angle, which can result in angle closure. Neovascularization of the angle may also occur after radiation therapy for intraocular tumors.

The most common cause of glaucoma associated with primary or metastatic tumors of the ciliary body is direct invasion of the anterior chamber angle. This glaucoma can be exacerbated by anterior segment hemorrhage and inflammation, which further obstruct aqueous outflow. Necrotic tumor and tumor-laden macrophages may cause obstruction of the trabecular meshwork and result in a secondary OAG. Tumors causing a secondary glaucoma in adults include uveal melanoma and melanocytoma (Figs 4-12, 4-13),

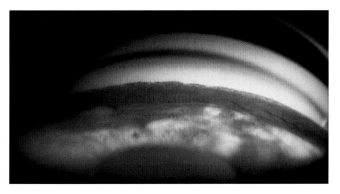

Figure 4-12   Goniophotograph of ciliary body melanoma in the anterior chamber angle. *(Courtesy of Wallace L. M. Alward, MD. From the* Iowa Glaucoma Curriculum *[curriculum.iowaglaucoma.org]. © The University of Iowa.)*

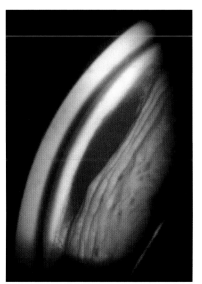

Figure 4-13   Goniophotograph of ciliary body melanocytoma in the anterior chamber angle. *(Courtesy of Wallace L. M. Alward, MD. From the* Iowa Glaucoma Curriculum *[curriculum .iowaglaucoma.org]. © The University of Iowa.)*

metastatic carcinoma, lymphoma, and leukemia. In children, tumors associated with glaucoma include retinoblastoma, juvenile xanthogranuloma, and medulloepithelioma.

Grostern RJ, Brown SVL. Glaucoma associated with intraocular tumors. In: Higginbotham E, Lee D, eds. *Management of Difficult Glaucomas.* Boston: Butterworth Heinemann; 2004: 343–351.

Shields CL, Materin MA, Shields JA, Gershenbaum E, Singh AD, Smith A. Factors associated with elevated intraocular pressure in eyes with iris melanoma. *Br J Ophthalmol.* 2001;85(6): 666–669.

Ocular Inflammation and Secondary Glaucoma

Inflammatory, or uveitic, glaucoma is a secondary glaucoma that often combines components of open-angle and angle-closure disease. In individuals with uveitis, elevated IOP may be caused by a variety of mechanisms; appropriate therapy depends on the etiology:

- edema of the trabecular meshwork
- endothelial cell dysfunction of the trabecular meshwork
- fibrin and inflammatory cells blocking outflow through the trabecular meshwork or Schlemm canal
- corticosteroid-induced reduction in outflow through the trabecular meshwork
- PAS blocking outflow
- prostaglandin-mediated breakdown of the blood–aqueous barrier

Most cases of anterior uveitis are idiopathic, but uveitides commonly associated with open-angle inflammatory glaucoma include Fuchs heterochromic uveitis (Fuchs heterochromic iridocyclitis), herpes zoster iridocyclitis, herpes simplex keratouveitis, toxoplasmosis, juvenile idiopathic arthritis, and pars planitis. See also BCSC Section 9, *Uveitis and Ocular Inflammation.*

The presence of KPs suggests anterior uveitis as the cause of IOP elevation. Gonioscopic evaluation may reveal subtle trabecular meshwork precipitates. Occasionally, PAS or posterior synechiae with iris bombé may develop, resulting in angle closure.

The treatment of inflammatory glaucoma is complicated by the fact that corticosteroid therapy may increase IOP, likely by increasing outflow resistance, but possibly by improving aqueous production as well. Miotic agents should be avoided in patients with anterior uveitis, because they may exacerbate the inflammation and cause formation of posterior synechiae. Prostaglandin analogues may exacerbate inflammation in some eyes with uveitis and herpetic keratitis; however, some patients may benefit from their IOP-lowering effects without increased inflammation.

Some uveitis patients may have low IOP. The etiology is unclear but may be related to a prostaglandin-mediated increase in uveoscleral outflow. Hyposecretion of aqueous humor (particularly if ciliary body detachment is present) has often been assumed to be the etiology for low IOP but has not been confirmed, as aqueous flow currently cannot be measured in the presence of uveitis.

Glaucomatocyclitic crisis

First described by Posner and Schlossman in 1948, glaucomatocyclitic crisis (also known as *Posner-Schlossman syndrome*) is an uncommon form of open-angle inflammatory glaucoma characterized by acute, unilateral episodes of markedly elevated IOP accompanied by a low-grade anterior chamber inflammation. This condition most frequently affects middle-aged persons, who usually present with unilateral blurred vision and mild ocular pain. The anterior uveitis is mild, with few KPs, which are small, discrete, and round and which usually resolve spontaneously within a few weeks. On gonioscopy, KPs may be seen on the trabecular meshwork, suggesting a "trabeculitis." The elevated IOP may range between 40 and 50 mm Hg, and corneal edema may be present. In between episodes, the IOP usually returns to normal, but with increasing numbers of episodes, a chronic secondary glaucoma may develop.

The etiology of glaucomatocyclitic crisis remains unknown, but theories include various infections (eg, herpes simplex virus) and autoimmune disease. Recurrent attacks of acute angle-closure glaucoma have been mistaken for this condition. In some cases in which glaucomatocyclitic crisis was initially diagnosed, cytomegalovirus DNA was subsequently detected in the aqueous humor by polymerase chain reaction (see BCSC Section 9, *Uveitis and Ocular Inflammation,* for discussion of cytomegalovirus). Distinguishing glaucomatocyclitic crisis from cytomegalovirus is important, because specific antiviral therapy for cytomegalovirus is available.

During a glaucomatocyclitic crisis, treatment should be initiated to control IOP and reduce inflammation. Topical (eg, β-blockers) and often oral (eg, carbonic anhydrase inhibitors) ocular hypotensive medications are used to reduce IOP. Prostaglandin analogues may exacerbate the condition. Topical corticosteroids and topical and/or oral nonsteroidal anti-inflammatory medications (eg, indomethacin) may be of benefit. There is no evidence that long-term suppressive therapy with topical nonsteroidal anti-inflammatory agents or corticosteroids is effective in preventing attacks.

Fuchs heterochromic uveitis

Fuchs heterochromic uveitis (also called *Fuchs heterochromic iridocyclitis*) is a relatively rare, insidious, and chronic form of uveitis that is typically unilateral. There is no race or sex predilection, and it often manifests in young to middle adulthood. It is characterized by iris heterochromia, low-grade anterior chamber inflammation, posterior subcapsular cataracts, and secondary OAG. The heterochromia is due to loss of iris pigment in the affected eye, which is usually hypochromic in dark eyes and hyperchromic in light eyes. The low-grade inflammation is often accompanied by small, stellate, pancorneal KPs. Despite the low-grade inflammation, these patients are classically asymptomatic and present with a nonhyperemic eye.

Secondary OAG occurs in approximately 15% of patients with this disease. On gonioscopy, multiple fine vessels may be viewed crossing the trabecular meshwork (Fig 4-14). These vessels are usually not accompanied by a fibrous membrane and typically do not result in PAS formation and secondary angle closure, although in rare cases the neovascularization may be progressive. The vessels are fragile and may cause an anterior chamber hemorrhage, either spontaneously or with trauma. A classic finding is anterior chamber hemorrhage after a paracentesis during ocular surgery (Amsler sign).

Treatment of Fuchs heterochromic uveitis is directed at controlling the IOP with topical ocular hypotensive medications. IOP control may be difficult, and the IOP does not necessarily correspond with the degree of inflammation. Corticosteroids are generally

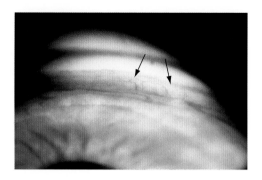

Figure 4-14 Fuchs heterochromic uveitis. The goniophotograph shows fine vessels *(arrows)* crossing the trabecular meshwork. This neovascularization is not accompanied by a fibrovascular membrane and does not result in peripheral anterior synechiae formation and secondary angle closure. *(Courtesy of Steven T. Simmons, MD.)*

not effective in treating the low-grade chronic inflammation, and their use could elevate the IOP. Recent studies suggest that rubella virus infection may be the underlying etiology of this condition.

Birnbaum AD, Tessler HH, Schultz KL, et al. Epidemiologic relationship between Fuchs heterochromic iridocyclitis and the United States rubella vaccination program. *Am J Ophthalmol.* 2007;144(3):424–428.

Elevated Episcleral Venous Pressure

Episcleral venous pressure (EVP) is an important factor in the determination of IOP. Normal EVP ranges between 6 and 9 mm Hg, depending on the measurement technique used. Elevated EVP may occur because of a variety of clinical entities that either result in obstruction of venous outflow or involve arteriovenous malformations (Table 4-3).

Patients may note a chronic red eye without ocular discomfort, itching, or discharge. Occasionally, a distant history of a significant head trauma may suggest the cause of a carotid-cavernous sinus (high-flow) or dural (low-flow) fistula. However, most cases are idiopathic, and some may be familial. Clinically, patients with elevated EVP present with tortuous, dilated episcleral veins (Fig 4-15). These vascular abnormalities may be unilateral or bilateral. Gonioscopy often reveals blood in the Schlemm canal (see Chapter 3, Fig 3-5). In rare instances, signs of ocular ischemia or venous stasis may be present. Sudden, severe carotid-cavernous fistulas may be accompanied by proptosis and other orbital

---

Table 4-3 Causes of Elevated Episcleral Venous Pressure

Arteriovenous malformations
 Arteriovenous fistula
  Dural
   Carotid-cavernous sinus
  Orbital varix
  Sturge-Weber syndrome

Venous obstruction
 Retrobulbar tumor
 Thyroid eye disease

Superior vena cava syndrome

Idiopathic (may be familial)

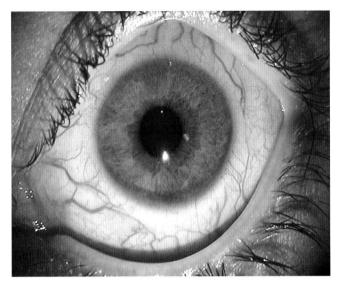

Figure 4-15 Prominent episcleral vessels in a patient with idiopathic elevated episcleral venous pressure. *(Courtesy of Keith Barton, MD.)*

or neurologic signs. Patients should undergo magnetic resonance imaging or angiography to rule out a vascular malformation. If these tests fail to show an abnormality and the clinical suspicion is high, traditional angiography with neuroradiologic intervention (eg, coiling of fistula) should be considered when the benefits to the patient outweigh the risks.

Topical ocular hypotensive medications, particularly those that reduce aqueous production, may be effective in some patients. Due to the etiology of the condition, laser trabeculoplasty is likely not effective. Glaucoma filtering surgery may be indicated. However, given the risk of a ciliochoroidal effusion or suprachoroidal hemorrhage, prophylactic sclerotomies or scleral windows may be necessary.

Trauma and Surgery

Nonpenetrating, or blunt, trauma to the eye causes a variety of anterior segment conditions that may lead to secondary glaucoma:

- inflammation
- hyphema
- angle recession
- lens subluxation (see Chapter 5, ectopia lentis)

These findings, particularly when in combination, often lead to elevated IOP initially after trauma. This elevation tends to be brief but may be protracted and result in glaucomatous optic nerve damage.

Siderosis or *chalcosis* from a retained intraocular metallic foreign body in penetrating or perforating injuries may lead to chronic OAG. Chemical injuries, particularly those involving alkali, may cause acute secondary glaucoma as a result of inflammation, shrinkage of scleral collagen, release of chemical mediators such as prostaglandins, direct damage to the anterior chamber angle, or compromised anterior uveal circulation. Recurrent inflammation or damage to the trabecular meshwork may progress to glaucoma over months or years after a chemical injury.

Traumatic hyphema

The risk of elevated IOP after a traumatic hyphema is increased with recurrent hemorrhage, or rebleeding. The average reported frequency of rebleeding after an initial hyphema is 5%–10%, but it varies significantly with different study populations. Rebleeding usually occurs within 3–7 days of the initial hyphema and may be related to normal clot retraction and lysis. In general, the larger the hyphema, the higher the incidence of increased IOP, although small hemorrhages may also be associated with marked elevation of IOP, particularly when the angle is already compromised. Increased IOP occurs as a result of obstruction of the trabecular meshwork with red blood cells (RBCs), inflammatory cells, debris, and fibrin, as well as from direct injury to the trabecular meshwork from the blunt trauma. Careful gonioscopic examination in individuals with blunt trauma may reveal a subtle hyphema. In addition to glaucomatous damage, prolonged IOP elevation in an eye with a hyphema increases the risk of corneal blood staining (Fig 4-16).

Individuals with sickle cell hemoglobinopathies have an increased risk of elevated IOP following hyphema and are more susceptible to the development of optic neuropathy. Normal RBCs pass through the trabecular meshwork without difficulty. However, in the sickle cell hemoglobinopathies (including sickle cell trait), the low pH of the aqueous humor causes the RBCs to sickle and become rigid. These more rigid cells become trapped in the trabecular meshwork, and even small amounts of sickle-shaped RBCs may cause marked elevations in IOP. In addition, the optic nerves of patients with sickle cell disease are much more sensitive to elevated IOP and are prone to development of anterior ischemic optic neuropathy and central retinal artery occlusion, as a result of compromised microvascular perfusion.

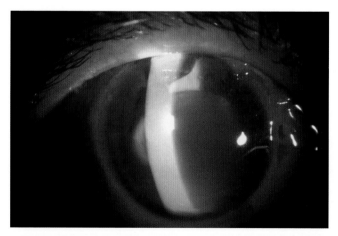

Figure 4-16 Corneal blood staining following trauma. Note the area of layered heme in the inferior angle. *(Courtesy of Wallace L. M. Alward, MD. From the Iowa Glaucoma Curriculum [curriculum.iowaglaucoma .org]. © The University of Iowa.)*

In general, the patient with an uncomplicated hyphema should be managed conservatively, with an eye shield, limited activity, and head elevation. Topical and oral corticosteroids may reduce associated inflammation, although their effect on rebleeding is debatable. If significant ciliary spasm or photophobia occurs, cycloplegic agents may be helpful, but they have no proven benefit for prevention of rebleeding. Oral administration of aminocaproic acid has been shown to reduce rebleeding in some studies. However, this has not been confirmed in all studies, and systemic adverse effects, such as hypotension, syncope, abdominal pain, and nausea, can be significant. Also, discontinuation of aminocaproic acid may be associated with clot lysis and additional IOP elevation.

Treatment of elevated IOP in patients with hyphema includes ocular hypotensive agents, particularly aqueous suppressants, and hyperosmotic agents. It has been suggested that patients with sickle cell hemoglobinopathies avoid carbonic anhydrase inhibitors, because these agents may increase the sickling tendency in the anterior chamber by further lowering the pH; however, this relationship has not been firmly established. Physicians should be aware that the use of systemic carbonic anhydrase inhibitors and hyperosmotic agents may induce a sickle crisis in susceptible individuals who are significantly dehydrated. Adrenergic agonists with significant α_1-agonist effects (apraclonidine, dipivefrin, epinephrine) should also be avoided in patients with sickle cell disease, because of the potential for anterior segment vasoconstriction with their use. Parasympathomimetic agents should be avoided in all patients with traumatic hyphema.

For patients with sickle cell disease, clinicians should have a lower threshold for surgical intervention, given these patients' increased risk of optic neuropathy from elevated IOP. In young children, vision obstruction by the hyphema or corneal blood staining may justify early surgical intervention to reduce the risk of amblyopia. If surgery for elevated IOP becomes necessary, an anterior chamber irrigation is commonly performed first. If a total hyphema is present, pupillary block may occur, and an iridectomy is helpful at the time of the washout. If the IOP remains uncontrolled, filtering surgery may be required. Some surgeons prefer to perform glaucoma filtering surgery with the anterior chamber washout in order to obtain immediate control of IOP, relieve any pupillary block, and reduce the risk of elevated IOP in the future from damage to the trabecular meshwork.

Campagna JA. Traumatic hyphema: current strategies. *Focal Points: Clinical Modules for Ophthalmologists.* San Francisco: American Academy of Ophthalmology; 2007, module 10.

Gharaibeh A, Savage HI, Scherer RW, Goldberg MF, Lindsley K. Medical interventions for traumatic hyphema. *Cochrane Database Syst Rev.* 2013;12:CD005431. Accessed September 22, 2015.

Hemolytic and ghost cell glaucoma

Hemolytic glaucoma, ghost cell glaucoma, or both may develop after a vitreous hemorrhage. In *hemolytic glaucoma,* hemoglobin-laden macrophages block the trabecular meshwork. Red-tinged cells are seen floating in the anterior chamber, and the trabecular meshwork may appear reddish brown. In *ghost cell glaucoma,* degenerated RBCs (ghost cells) obstruct the trabecular meshwork.

Ghost cells are small, khaki-colored RBCs that have lost their intracellular hemoglobin (Fig 4-17). They are less pliable than normal RBCs; thus, they obstruct the trabecular

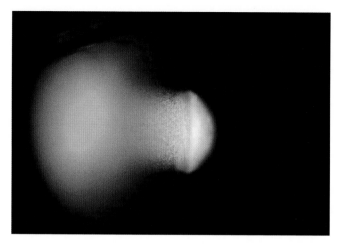

Figure 4-17 Ghost cell glaucoma: the classic appearance of ghost cells in the anterior chamber. These small, khaki-colored cells can become layered, as occurs in a hyphema or hypopyon. *(Courtesy of Ron Gross, MD.)*

meshwork and cause elevated IOP. RBCs degenerate within 1–3 months after a vitreous hemorrhage. They gain access to the anterior chamber through a disrupted hyaloid face, which can occur from previous surgery (pars plana vitrectomy, cataract extraction, or capsulotomy) or trauma or spontaneously.

Patients with ghost cell glaucoma typically present with elevated IOP and a history of or current vitreous hemorrhage from trauma, surgery, or preexisting retinal disease. The IOP may be markedly elevated, with accompanying corneal edema. The anterior chamber may contain degenerated RBCs. The cellular reaction is often out of proportion to the aqueous flare, and the conjunctiva tends not to be inflamed unless the IOP is markedly elevated. On gonioscopy, the angle appears normal except for possible layering of ghost cells in the inferior angle. A long-standing vitreous hemorrhage may be present, with characteristic khaki coloration and clumps of extracellular pigmentation from degenerated hemoglobin.

Hemolytic glaucoma and ghost cell glaucoma generally resolve once the hemorrhage has cleared. Medical therapy with aqueous suppressants is the preferred initial approach. If medical therapy fails to control the IOP, some patients may require anterior chamber irrigation, pars plana vitrectomy, and/or incisional glaucoma surgery. When a collection of RBCs or ghost cells is present in the vitreous, a pars plana vitrectomy is likely necessary for IOP control.

Traumatic, or angle-recession, glaucoma

Angle recession is a common finding after blunt trauma and involves a tear between the longitudinal and circular fibers of the ciliary body. It is important to note that angle recession is not necessarily associated with immediate IOP elevation and glaucoma; however, it is a sign of probable damage to the underlying trabecular meshwork. Traumatic glaucoma is chronic and usually unilateral and may occur immediately after the ocular trauma or months to years later. It resembles POAG in presentation and clinical course but can be distinguished by its classic gonioscopic findings (Figs 4-18, 4-19):

- widening of the ciliary body band
- absent or torn iris processes
- white, glistening scleral spur
- irregular and dark pigmentation in the angle
- PAS at the border of the recession

Traumatic glaucoma should be considered in a patient with unilateral IOP elevation. The patient's history may reveal the contributing incident; often, however, this has been forgotten. Examination may reveal findings consistent with previous trauma, such as corneal scars, iris injury, abnormalities in the angle, focal anterior subcapsular cataracts, and phacodonesis. Comparing gonioscopic findings in the affected eye to those in the fellow eye may help the clinician identify areas of recession.

More extensive angle recession is associated with a greater reduction in outflow facility and an increased risk of glaucoma. However, even with substantial angle recession,

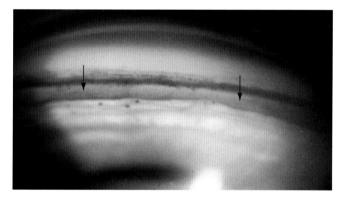

Figure 4-18 Goniophotograph of angle recession. Angle recession occurs when the ciliary body is torn, usually between the longitudinal and circular fibers of the ciliary body, resulting in a deepened angle recess *(arrows)*. The dark circular deposits located on the peripheral iris represent old heme. *(Reproduced from Alward WLM, Longmuir RA. Color Atlas of Gonioscopy. 2nd ed. San Francisco: American Academy of Ophthalmology; 2008:89. Fig 9-50.)*

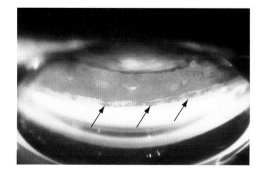

Figure 4-19 Typical gonioscopic appearance of angle recession. Torn iris processes *(arrows)*, a whitened and increasingly visible scleral spur, and a localized depression in the trabecular meshwork are shown. *(Courtesy of Steven T. Simmons, MD.)*

this risk is not high. Although the risk of developing glaucoma decreases appreciably after several years, it is still present even 25 years or more following injury. In a significant proportion (up to 50%) of fellow eyes, elevated IOP may occur, suggesting that eyes with traumatic glaucoma may be predisposed to OAG. Because it is not possible to predict which eyes will develop glaucoma, all eyes with angle recession and their fellow eyes should be monitored annually.

The treatment of traumatic glaucoma is often initiated with aqueous suppressants, prostaglandin analogues, and α_2-adrenergic agonists. Miotics may be useful, but paradoxical responses of increased IOP may occur. Laser trabeculoplasty has a limited role and a reduced likelihood of success. Incisional glaucoma surgery may be required in order to control the IOP in patients not responding to medical therapy.

Surgery

Conventional surgical procedures such as cataract extraction, trabeculectomy, tube shunt implantation, and penetrating keratoplasty (see also the following subsection) may be followed by an increase in IOP. Similarly, laser surgery—including trabeculoplasty, iridotomy, and posterior capsulotomy—may be complicated by posttreatment IOP elevation. Although the IOP may rise as high as 50 mm Hg or more, these elevations are usually transient, lasting from a few hours to a few days. The exact mechanism is not always known. However, the presence of inflammatory cells, RBCs, and debris; pigment release; mechanical deformation of the trabecular meshwork; and angle closure may all be implicated.

In addition, agents used as adjuncts to intraocular surgery or postoperative treatment (corticosteroids) may cause secondary IOP elevation. For example, the injection of viscoelastic substances such as sodium hyaluronate into the anterior chamber may result in a transient and possibly severe postoperative increase in IOP. Dispersive viscoelastic agents, especially in higher-molecular-weight forms, may be more likely to cause an increase in IOP than cohesive viscoelastics.

Postoperative IOP elevation, even over a short period, can cause considerable damage to the optic nerve in susceptible individuals. Eyes with preexisting glaucoma are particularly at risk of further damage; thus, it is extremely important to monitor IOP soon after conventional or laser surgery. If a substantial rise in IOP occurs, IOP-lowering therapy may be required, including the use of topical β-blockers, α_2-adrenergic agonists, or carbonic anhydrase inhibitors. If postoperative inflammation is present, prostaglandin analogues may be deferred until the inflammation has resolved. Persistent IOP elevation may require filtering surgery.

The implantation of an intraocular lens (IOL) can lead to a variety of secondary glaucomas, including the following:

- uveitis-glaucoma-hyphema syndrome
- secondary pigmentary glaucoma
- pseudophakic pupillary block (see Chapter 5)

Uveitis-glaucoma-hyphema (UGH) syndrome is a secondary inflammatory glaucoma classically caused by chafing of the iris by a malpositioned or rotated anterior chamber IOL.

This condition can also occur following implantation of a posterior chamber or suture-fixated IOL. UGH syndrome often results in chronic inflammation, elevated IOP, and recurrent hyphemas, as well as cystoid macular edema and secondary iris neovascularization. Gonioscopy and ultrasound biomicroscopy may be helpful in revealing the IOL's exact position in relation to the iris and ciliary body. Persistent or recurrent cases often require IOL repositioning or IOL exchange, which can be technically challenging because of possible synechiae and/or an open posterior capsule. This syndrome may be mimicked in patients with neovascularization of the internal lip of a corneoscleral wound, which may result in recurrent spontaneous hyphemas and elevated IOP. Argon laser ablation of the vessels may successfully resolve these cases.

Secondary glaucoma is a common complication after penetrating keratoplasty (PKP) and occurs with greater frequency in aphakic and pseudophakic patients and after a second graft. Wound distortion of the trabecular meshwork and progressive angle closure are the most common causes of glaucoma after PKP. Attempts to minimize these changes with different-sized donor grafts, peripheral iridectomies, and surgical repair of the iris sphincter have only been partially successful. Procedures such as lamellar or endothelial keratoplasty (EK) may have a lower risk of elevated IOP, although the air bubbles used with EK may cause secondary angle closure. Long-term topical corticosteroid use after PKP is another potential cause of elevated IOP and secondary glaucoma in these patients. See BCSC Section 8, *External Disease and Cornea,* for further discussion of PKP.

Jarstad JS, Hardwig PW. Intraocular hemorrhage from wound neovascularization years after anterior segment surgery (Swan syndrome). *Can J Ophthalmol.* 1987;22(5):271–275.

Schwartz Syndrome (Schwartz-Matsuo Syndrome)

Individuals with a rhegmatogenous retinal detachment typically have lower IOP, presumably because of increased outflow of fluid through the exposed retinal pigment epithelium. Schwartz was the first to describe elevated IOP associated with a rhegmatogenous retinal detachment. Matsuo later demonstrated the presence of photoreceptor outer segments in the aqueous humor of patients with rhegmatogenous retinal detachments. The postulated mechanism of IOP elevation is the liberation of photoreceptor outer segments, which migrate through the retinal tear into the anterior chamber and impede aqueous outflow through the trabecular meshwork. The photoreceptor segments may be mistaken for an anterior chamber inflammatory reaction or pigment. The IOP tends to normalize after successful surgery to reattach the retina.

Drugs and Glaucoma

Corticosteroid-induced glaucoma is an OAG caused by prolonged use of topical, periocular, intravitreal, inhaled, or oral corticosteroids. It mimics POAG in its presentation and clinical course. Approximately one-third of the population without glaucoma demonstrates an IOP elevation of between 6 and 15 mm Hg in response to corticosteroids, and only a small percentage (4%–6%) has a significant IOP elevation of more than 15 mm Hg. A high percentage (up to 95%) of patients with POAG demonstrate a response to topical corticosteroids. The type and potency of the agent, the means and frequency of its administration, and the susceptibility of the patient all affect the timing and extent of the IOP rise. Risk factors for corticosteroid-induced glaucoma include a history of POAG, a first-degree relative with POAG, very young age (<6 years) or older age, connective tissue disease, type 1 diabetes mellitus, and myopia. The elevated IOP is a result of increased resistance to aqueous outflow in the trabecular meshwork. See also BCSC Section 9, *Uveitis and Ocular Inflammation,* for further discussion of corticosteroids.

Corticosteroid-induced glaucoma may develop within weeks, months, or years of the drug's use; thus, IOP should be monitored regularly in patients receiving these agents. In general, the potency of the anti-inflammatory glucocorticoid activity of a particular drug parallels its ocular hypertensive potency. For example, some corticosteroid preparations, such as fluorometholone, rimexolone, medrysone, or loteprednol, are less likely to raise IOP than are prednisolone, dexamethasone, or difluprednate (see Table 16-15 in BCSC Section 2, *Fundamentals and Principles of Ophthalmology*). However, even weaker corticosteroids or lower concentrations of stronger drugs can raise IOP in susceptible individuals. A corticosteroid-induced rise in IOP may cause glaucomatous optic nerve damage in some patients.

The cause of the elevation in IOP may be related to an underlying ocular disease, such as anterior uveitis, as opposed to corticosteroid use. After the corticosteroid is discontinued, the IOP usually decreases with a time course similar to or slightly longer than that of the onset of elevation. However, unmasked POAG or secondary open-angle inflammatory glaucoma may remain.

IOP may also become elevated in patients who have excessive levels of endogenous corticosteroids (eg, Cushing syndrome). When the corticosteroid-producing tumor or hyperplastic tissue is excised, IOP generally returns to normal.

Periocular injection of corticosteroid may result in elevated IOP. Medical therapy may lower the IOP, but some patients require excision of the depot of corticosteroid or glaucoma surgery.

Intravitreal corticosteroid injection may be associated with transient elevations in IOP in more than 50% of patients. Up to 25% of these patients may require topical medications to control IOP, and 1%–2% may require incisional glaucoma surgery. In contrast, intravitreal implants that release corticosteroid are frequently associated with elevated IOP, often requiring patients to undergo incisional glaucoma surgery for IOP control. Surgical treatment has a high success rate in lowering IOP in these patients; laser trabeculoplasty may also be of benefit.

Cycloplegic drugs can increase IOP in individuals with open angles. Routine dilation for ophthalmoscopy may increase IOP; those at greater risk include patients with POAG, pseudoexfoliation syndrome, or pigment dispersion syndrome, as well as those receiving miotic therapy.

Intravitreal injection of antivascular endothelial growth factor (anti-VEGF) is a common treatment for exudative macular degeneration. Intravitreal injection may result in a transient rise in IOP, and repeated injections, over time, may result in sustained IOP elevation. The etiology of the elevated IOP is unknown, but theories include increased inflammation and injury to or mechanical blockage of the trabecular meshwork.

Epstein DL, Allingham RR, Schuman JS, eds. *Chandler and Grant's Glaucoma.* 4th ed. Baltimore: Williams & Wilkins; 1997.

Shields MB, Allingham RR, Damji K. *Shields' Textbook of Glaucoma.* 5th ed. Philadelphia: Lippincott Williams & Wilkins; 2004.

SooHoo JR, Seibold LK, Kahook MY. The link between intravitreal antivascular endothelial growth factor injections and glaucoma. *Curr Opin Ophthalmol.* 2014;25(2):127–133.

CLINICAL TRIAL 4-1

Collaborative Initial Glaucoma Treatment Study (CIGTS) Essentials

Purpose: To determine whether patients with newly diagnosed open-angle glaucoma (OAG) are better treated by initial treatment with medications or by immediate filtering surgery.

Participants: 607 patients with OAG (primary, pigmentary, or pseudoexfoliation) recruited between 1993 and 1997.

Study design: Multicenter randomized controlled clinical trial comparing initial medical therapy with initial surgical therapy for OAG.

Results: Although IOP was lower in the surgery group, initial medical and initial surgical therapy resulted in similar visual field outcomes after up to 9 years of follow-up. Early visual acuity loss was greater in the surgery group, but the differences between groups converged over time. Also, cataracts were more common in the surgery group. At the 8-year follow-up examination, substantial worsening ($\geq$3 dB) of visual field mean deviation from baseline was found in 21.3% of the initial surgery group and 25.5% of the initial medical group. Patients with worse baseline visual fields were less likely to progress if treated with trabeculectomy first. Patients with diabetes mellitus were more likely to progress if treated initially with surgery.

The quality of life (QOL) reported by the 2 treatment groups was similar. The most persistent QOL finding was a greater number of symptoms reported at a higher frequency by the surgery group.

The overall rate of progression of OAG was lower in CIGTS than in many clinical trials, possibly because of more aggressive IOP-lowering goals and the stage of the disease. Individualized target IOPs were determined according to a formula that accounted for baseline IOP and visual field loss. Over the course of follow-up, IOP in the medical therapy group averaged 17–18 mm Hg (IOP reduction of approximately 38%), whereas IOP in the surgery group averaged 14–15 mm Hg (IOP reduction of approximately 46%). IOP fluctuation was a risk factor for progression in the medically treated group but not the surgically treated group. The rate of cataract removal was greater in the surgically treated group.

CLINICAL TRIAL 4-2

Ocular Hypertension Treatment Study (OHTS) Essentials

Purpose: To evaluate the safety and efficacy of topical ocular hypotensive medications in preventing or delaying the onset of visual field loss and/or optic nerve damage in participants with ocular hypertension.

Participants: 1637 patients with ocular hypertension recruited between 1994 and 1996.

Study design: Multicenter randomized controlled clinical trial comparing observation and medical therapy for ocular hypertension.

Results 2002: Topical ocular hypotensive medication was effective in delaying or preventing the onset of primary open-angle glaucoma (POAG). The incidence of glaucoma was lower in the medication group than in the observation group (4.4% vs 9.5%, respectively) at 60 months' follow-up. No increase in adverse events was detected in the medication group.

The 5-year risk of developing POAG was associated with the following baseline factors: older age (22% increase in relative risk per decade), larger vertical and horizontal cup–disc ratios (32% and 27% increases in relative risk per 0.1 increase, respectively), higher pattern standard deviation (22% increase in relative risk per 0.2 dB increase), and higher baseline IOP (10% increase in relative risk per 1 mm Hg increase). Central corneal thickness (CCT) was found to be a powerful predictor for the development of POAG (81% increase in relative risk for every 40 μm thinner). The corneas in OHTS participants were thicker than those in the general population, and African American participants had thinner corneas than others in the study.

Results 2007: The OHTS prediction model for the development of POAG was independently validated in the European Glaucoma Prevention Study.

Results 2010: Topical ocular hypotensive medication was initiated in the original observation group after 7.5 years (median) without medication, and medication was continued for 5.5 years thereafter. Participants in the original medication group continued topical ocular hypotensive medications for a median of 13 years. The proportion of participants who developed POAG was 0.22 in the original observation group and 0.16 in the original medication group. The primary purpose of the follow-up study was to determine whether delaying treatment resulted in a persistently increased risk of conversion to glaucoma, even after the initiation of therapy. Although the two groups diverged with respect to the development of glaucoma during the original study period (when the observation group did not receive treatment), there was no further divergence in the Kaplan-Meier curves after both groups received IOP-lowering treatment.

CLINICAL TRIAL 4-3

Early Manifest Glaucoma Trial (EMGT) Essentials

Purpose: To evaluate the effectiveness of lowering IOP in patients with early, newly detected OAG.

Participants: Patients 50 to 80 years of age with newly diagnosed OAG and early glaucomatous visual field loss were identified mainly through a population-based screening of more than 44,000 residents of Malmö and Helsingborg, Sweden. Exclusion criteria were advanced visual field loss; mean IOP greater than 30 mm Hg or any IOP greater than 35 mm Hg; and visual acuity less than 0.5 (20/40). Two hundred fifty-five patients were randomized between 1993 and 1997.

Study design: Multicenter randomized controlled clinical trial comparing observation and treatment with betaxolol and argon laser trabeculoplasty for OAG.

Results: At 6 years, 62% of untreated patients showed progression, whereas 45% of treated patients progressed. On average, treatment reduced IOP by 25%. In a univariate analysis, risk factors for progression included no IOP-lowering treatment, older age, higher IOP, pseudoexfoliation syndrome, more advanced visual field loss, and bilateral glaucoma. In multivariate analyses, the risk of progression with IOP-lowering treatment was reduced by half (HR = 0.50; 95% confidence interval, 0.35–0.71). Each mm Hg of IOP lowering decreased the risk of glaucomatous progression by 10%. Risk factors for progression included higher baseline IOP, older age, pseudoexfoliation syndrome, bilateral disease, worse mean deviation, and frequent disc hemorrhages. IOP fluctuation was not found to be a significant risk factor.

In the observation group, the rate of visual field progression was most rapid in the subgroup of patients with pseudoexfoliation syndrome and slowest in those with baseline IOPs within the normal range.

CLINICAL TRIAL 4-4

Advanced Glaucoma Intervention Study (AGIS) Essentials

Purpose: To compare the clinical outcomes of 2 treatment sequences: argon laser trabeculoplasty–trabeculectomy–trabeculectomy (ATT) and trabeculectomy–argon laser trabeculoplasty–trabeculectomy (TAT).

Participants: 789 eyes of 591 patients with medically uncontrolled OAG recruited from 1988 to 1992.

Study design: Multicenter randomized controlled clinical trial comparing 2 treatment sequences (ATT and TAT) for patients with OAG uncontrolled with medical therapy.

(Continued on next page)

(continued)

Results

AGIS 4 and AGIS 13: Black patients treated with the ATT sequence had a lower combined visual acuity and visual field loss than those treated with the TAT sequence. White patients had a lower combined visual acuity and visual field loss at 7 years if initially treated with the TAT sequence. In the initial follow-up period, white patients in the TAT group had greater visual acuity loss than those in the ATT group; by 7 years, this loss was similar.

AGIS 5: Encapsulated blebs were slightly more common in patients with prior argon laser trabeculoplasty (ALT), but this difference was not statistically significant. The mean IOP at the 4-week postoperative visit was higher in eyes with encapsulated blebs than in those without; with resumption of medical therapy, eyes with and without encapsulated blebs had similar IOPs after 1 year.

AGIS 6: Visual function scores improved after cataract surgery. Adjustment for cataract did not alter the findings of previous AGIS studies.

AGIS 7: Lower IOP was associated with less visual field progression. Less visual field progression was noted for eyes with an average IOP of 14 mm Hg or less during the first 18 months after the first surgical intervention, and for eyes with IOP of 18 mm Hg or less for all study visits.

AGIS 8: Approximately half of the study patients developed cataract in the first 5 years of follow-up. Trabeculectomy increased the relative risk of cataract formation by 78%.

AGIS 9: Trabeculectomy retards the progression of glaucoma more effectively in white patients than in black patients. ALT was slightly more effective in blacks than in whites.

AGIS 10: Assessment of optic nerve findings showed good intraobserver but poor interobserver agreement.

AGIS 11: Reduced effectiveness of ALT was associated with younger age and higher IOP. The ineffectiveness of trabeculectomy was associated with younger age, higher IOP, diabetes mellitus, and postoperative complications (markedly elevated IOP and inflammation).

AGIS 12: Risk factors for sustained decrease of the visual field included better baseline visual fields, male sex, worse baseline visual acuity, and diabetes mellitus. Risk factors for sustained decrease in visual acuity included better baseline visual acuity, older age, and less formal education.

AGIS 14: In patients with visual field progression, a single 6-month confirmatory visual field test had a 72% probability of verifying a persistent defect. When the number of confirmatory visual field tests was increased from 1 to 2, the percentage of eyes that showed a persistent defect increased from 72% to 84%.

2009 AGIS Report: Intraocular pressure fluctuation was an independent predictor of progression of OAG in eyes with lower baseline IOPs, but not in those with higher baseline IOPs.

Most of the relevant findings from AGIS that reflect clinical practice are from post hoc analysis; thus, they may not fully take into account unmeasurable confounding factors and enrollment bias.

CHAPTER 5

Angle-Closure Glaucoma

Introduction

Angle closure refers to an anatomical configuration in which there is mechanical block-age of the trabecular meshwork by the peripheral iris. Anatomical alterations in anterior segment structures obstruct the iridocorneal drainage angle through apposition or conse-quent to the formation of peripheral anterior synechiae (PAS). Traditionally, angle closure is divided into 2 main categories: primary and secondary angle closure. BCSC Section 10 uses these traditional categories but also incorporates the definitions of primary angle closure presented in the European Glaucoma Society classification to reflect trends in the ophthalmologic literature. The European Glaucoma Society has classified primary angle closure as follows, based on the natural course of the disease: *primary angle-closure sus-pect (PACS)*, in which the eye has an increased anatomical risk of angle closure; *primary angle closure (PAC)*, in which trabecular meshwork damage or dysfunction is character-ized by PAS or elevated intraocular pressure (IOP); and *primary angle-closure glaucoma (PACG)*, which is characterized by PAS or elevated IOP and glaucomatous optic neuropa-thy (Table 5-1).

The worldwide prevalence of angle-closure glaucoma (ACG) is estimated to be 16 million. ACG is more common in females and in certain ethnic groups, such as par-ticular Asian populations and the Inuit. Prevalence rates in European and African popula-tions are generally lower; however, genetic heterogeneity can result in widely varying rates within populations of the same continent. ACG has been estimated to account for over 90% of blindness due to glaucoma in the Chinese population.

The angle-closure-related disorders are a diverse group of diseases. While the var-ious forms of angle closure are unified by the presence of PAS and/or iridotrabecular

Table 5-1 European Glaucoma Society Classification of Angle Closure

Stage	Definition
Primary angle-closure suspect (PACS)	Iridotrabecular contact >180° but no evidence of trabecular meshwork or optic nerve damage
Primary angle closure (PAC)	Iridotrabecular contact >180° with elevated IOP or PAS but no optic nerve damage
Primary angle-closure glaucoma (PACG)	PAC with glaucomatous optic neuropathy

IOP = intraocular pressure; PAS = peripheral anterior synechiae.

apposition, the mechanism of synechiae formation or iris apposition varies. Moreover, the clinical presentation of angle closure varies from the abrupt and dramatic onset of acute angle closure to the insidious and asymptomatic presentation of chronic disease.

In either presentation, acute or chronic, the physician must identify the anatomical changes within the angle and the underlying pathophysiology that has precipitated these changes in order to initiate the appropriate therapy. Early diagnosis and treatment of most forms of angle closure or narrowing can be invaluable, and sometimes curative. Accordingly, understanding the pathophysiology is essential if proper treatment is to be initiated. Also, screening patients at greatest risk for angle closure can be beneficial in reducing the number of patients who develop these diseases and in reducing the risk of blindness.

Primary and secondary angle closure are subdivided by the symptomatology, etiology, and duration of each of the diseases. In *primary* angle closure, there is no identifiable secondary pathologic condition; there is only an anatomical predisposition. In *secondary* angle closure, an identifiable pathologic cause, such as an intumescent lens, iris neovascularization, chronic inflammation, corneal endothelial migration, or epithelial ingrowth, initiates the angle closure.

Yip JL, Foster PJ. Ethnic differences in primary angle-closure glaucoma. *Curr Opin Ophthalmol.* 2006;17(2):175–180.

Pathogenesis and Pathophysiology of Angle Closure

The hallmark of angle closure is the apposition or adhesion of the peripheral iris to the trabecular meshwork. The portion of the anterior chamber angle affected by such apposition is "closed," and drainage of aqueous humor through the angle is reduced as a result. Such closure may be transient and intermittent (appositional) or permanent (synechial). These 2 forms of angle closure can be distinguished using indentation gonioscopy. The IOP becomes elevated as a result of the reduced aqueous outflow through the trabecular meshwork.

Conceptually, the mechanisms of angle closure fall into 2 categories (Table 5-2):

- mechanisms that push the iris forward from behind
- mechanisms that pull the iris forward into contact with the trabecular meshwork

In addition to these traditional descriptions of angle closure, more recent work has suggested that the dynamic changes in iris volume and water content normally occurring in the human eye are dysfunctional in patients with ACG and may play an important role in the pathogenesis of angle closure. Indeed, there is mounting evidence that dynamic features of the eye rather than its static anatomy contribute to ACG.

Quigley HA. The iris is a sponge: a cause of angle closure. *Ophthalmology.* 2010;117(1):1–2.

Pupillary Block

Pupillary block is the most frequent cause of angle closure. The pathophysiology of PAC is complex and not completely understood, but pupillary block is the underlying cause of most cases of this disease. The flow of aqueous from the posterior chamber through the pupil is impeded at the level of the lens–iris interface, and this obstruction creates a

Table 5-2 Underlying Mechanisms of Angle Closure

Iris pushed forward from behind, into the angle:
- pupillary block
- malignant glaucoma (aqueous misdirection)
- ciliary body swelling, inflammation, or cysts
- anteriorly located ciliary processes (plateau iris configuration/syndrome)
- choroidal swelling, serous or hemorrhagic choroidal detachments or effusions
- posterior segment tumors or space-occupying lesions (silicone oil, gas bubble)
- contracting retrolental tissue (persistent fetal vasculature, retinopathy of prematurity)
- anteriorly displaced lens
- encircling retinal bands/scleral buckles

Iris pulled forward into contact with the trabecular meshwork:
- contraction of inflammatory membrane or fibrovascular tissue
- migration of corneal endothelium (iridocorneal endothelial [ICE] syndrome)
- fibrous ingrowth
- epithelial ingrowth
- iris incarceration in traumatic wound or surgical incision

pressure gradient between the posterior and anterior chambers, causing the peripheral iris to bow forward against the trabecular meshwork (Chapter 1, Fig 1-1). Pupillary block is maximal when the pupil is in the mid-dilated position. In most cases of PACG, pupillary block results from anatomical factors at the lens–iris interface. Though rare, *absolute pupillary block* occurs when there is no movement of aqueous through the pupil as a result of 360° of posterior synechiae (secluded pupil). These posterior synechiae can form between the iris and the lens or, in an aphakic eye, between the iris and capsular remnants and/or the vitreous face. Pupillary block occurs when there is restricted movement of aqueous through the pupil because of iris contact with the lens, intraocular lens, capsular remnants, anterior hyaloid, or vitreous space–occupying substance (air, silicone oil). Pupillary block may be broken by an unobstructed peripheral iridectomy or iridotomy.

Lens-Induced Pupillary Block Angle-Closure Glaucoma

Intumescent or dislocated lenses (complete zonular dehiscence) may increase pupillary block and cause angle closure. Angle closure from an unusually large or intumescent lens is often referred to as *phacomorphic glaucoma* (see the subsection "Phacomorphic glaucoma" later in this chapter). With lens subluxation (partial zonular dehiscence), as in Marfan syndrome, pseudoexfoliation syndrome, or homocystinuria, pupillary block from the lens or vitreous may occur. Lens block describes an underlying mechanism of PAC, in which the lens's increased anterior-posterior excursion is due to weakened or lax zonular fibers. This zonular laxity allows the lens to move forward, increasing the relative resistance to aqueous flow through the pupil, which can increase pupillary block, inciting angle closure. The prone position may increase the tendency of the lens to move forward.

Angle Closure Without Pupillary Block

Angle closure may occur without pupillary block. Iridotrabecular apposition or synechiae formation can result from the iris and/or lens being pushed, rotated, or pulled forward for a variety of reasons, as outlined in Table 5-2. Each of these underlying mechanisms can usually be identified by a comprehensive examination, including gonioscopy. Many patients present with multiple underlying causes for their angle closure.

Iris-Induced Angle Closure

In iris-induced angle closure, the peripheral iris is the cause of the iridotrabecular apposition. Iris-induced angle closure can occur directly with developmental anomalies such as anterior cleavage abnormalities, in which the iris insertion into the scleral spur or meshwork is more anterior; a thick peripheral iris, which on dilatation "rolls" into the trabecular meshwork; and/or anteriorly displaced ciliary processes, which may secondarily rotate the peripheral iris forward (plateau iris) into the meshwork. Iris-induced angle closure also occurs in aniridia: the rudimentary iris leaflets present in aniridia rotate into the angle, resulting in secondary angle closure.

Primary Angle Closure

Risk Factors for Developing Primary Angle Closure

Race

The prevalence of PACG in patients older than 40 years varies greatly depending on race and ethnicity; for example, it is 0.1%–0.2% in blacks, 0.1%–0.6% in whites, 0.3% in the Japanese, 0.4%–1.4% in other East Asians, 2.1%–5.0% in the Inuit, and 2.3% in a mixed ethnic group in South Africa. Some of this variation in prevalence—for example, between whites and the Inuit—can be explained by differences in the biometric parameters (anterior chamber depth, axial length) of these groups; however, the increased prevalence of PACG in the Chinese and in other East Asian populations cannot be explained by biometric parameters alone. It has become increasingly clear that the burden of PACG is greater in Asian countries.

Bonomi L, Marchini G, Marraffa M, et al. Epidemiology of angle-closure glaucoma: prevalence, clinical types, and association with peripheral anterior chamber depth in the Egna-Neumarket Glaucoma Study. *Ophthalmology.* 2000;107(5):998–1003.

Dandona L, Dandona R, Mandal P, et al. Angle-closure glaucoma in an urban population in southern India: the Andhra Pradesh Eye Disease Study. *Ophthalmology.* 2000;107(9): 1710–1716.

Day AC, Baio G, Gazzard G, et al. The prevalence of primary angle closure glaucoma in European derived populations: a systematic review. *Br J Ophthalmol.* 2012;96(9): 1162–1167.

Foster PJ, Oen FT, Machin D, et al. The prevalence of glaucoma in Chinese residents of Singapore: a cross-sectional population survey of the Tanjong Pagar district. *Arch Ophthalmol.* 2000;118(8):1105–1111.

Quigley HA. Angle-closure glaucoma—simpler answers to complex mechanisms: LXVI Edward Jackson Memorial Lecture. *Am J Ophthalmol.* 2009;148(5):657–669.

Quigley HA, Broman AT. The number of people with glaucoma worldwide in 2010 and 2020. *Br J Ophthalmol.* 2006;90(3):262–267.

Ocular biometrics

Eyes that develop PAC tend to have small, "crowded" anterior segments and short axial lengths (ALs). The most important factors predisposing an eye to angle closure are a shallow anterior chamber, a thick lens, increased anterior curvature of the lens, a short AL, and a small corneal diameter and radius of curvature. An anterior chamber depth (ACD) of less than 2.5 mm predisposes patients to PAC; in fact, in most patients with PAC, the ACD is less than 2.1 mm. Improvements in ocular biometry techniques have allowed researchers to demonstrate a clear association between ACD and PAS. While primary PAS seem to be uncommon in eyes whose ACD is greater than 2.4 mm, there is a strong correlation of increasing PAS formation with an ACD of less than 2.4 mm. However, angle closure still occurs in eyes with deep anterior chambers in some cases.

The prevalence of PAC increases with each decade after 40 years of age. This has been explained by the increasing thickness and forward movement of the lens with age and the resultant increase in iridolenticular contact. PAC is rare in persons younger than 40 years, and the etiology of angle closure in young individuals is most often related to structural or developmental anomalies rather than pupillary block.

Aung T, Nolan WP, Machin D, et al. Anterior chamber depth and the risk of primary angle closure in 2 East Asian populations. *Arch Ophthalmol.* 2005;123(4):527–532.

Devereux JG, Foster PJ, Baasanhu J, et al. Anterior chamber depth measurement as a screening tool for primary angle-closure glaucoma in an East Asian population. *Arch Ophthalmol.* 2000;118(2):257–263.

Ritch R, Chang BM, Liebmann JM. Angle closure in younger patients. *Ophthalmology.* 2003;110(10):1880–1889.

Sex

Primary angle closure is 2 to 4 times more common in women than in men, irrespective of race. Studies assessing ocular biometry data have found that women tend to have smaller anterior segments and shorter ALs than men. These differences do not appear to be large enough to explain the gender predilection, however.

Family history

The incidence of PAC is increased in first-degree relatives of affected individuals. In whites, the prevalence of PAC in first-degree relatives has been reported to be between 1% and 12%, whereas results from a survey in a Chinese population showed that the risk was 6 times higher in patients with any family history. In the Inuit, the relative risk in patients with a positive family history is increased 3.5 times compared with the general Inuit population. These familial associations support a genetic influence in PAC. A recent genomewide association study reported the association of an *ABCC5* gene variant with reduced ACD and increased risk of PACG. A further study identified 3 loci associated with PACG.

Nongpiur ME, Khor CC, Jia H, et al. *ABCC5*, a gene that influences the anterior chamber depth, is associated with primary angle closure glaucoma. *PLoS Genet.* 2014;10(3): e1004089.

Vithana EN, Khor CC, Qiao C, et al. Genome-wide association analyses identify three new susceptibility loci for primary angle closure glaucoma. *Nat Genet.* 2012;44(10):1142–1146.

Refractive error

Primary angle closure occurs most commonly, but not exclusively, in patients with hyperopia, irrespective of race. Increasing rates of myopia, especially in Asia, have influenced the prevalence of this disease. Nonetheless, angle closure does occur in patients with significant myopia, underscoring the need to perform gonioscopy in all patients. Angle closure in a patient with high myopia should prompt the clinician to search for secondary mechanisms such as microspherophakia, plateau iris configuration, or phacomorphic closure related to nuclear sclerotic cataract.

Primary Angle-Closure Suspect

An eye termed *primary angle-closure suspect (PACS)* has an occludable, or narrow, anterior chamber angle but no overt signs of PAC (IOP elevation or PAS) or glaucomatous optic nerve damage. Thus, a narrow angle is not synonymous with a diagnosis of glaucoma, and the term is an anatomical description only. PACS eyes with shorter axial lengths are also at risk for PAC.

Only a small percentage of eyes with shallow anterior chambers develop PAC. Unfortunately, the predictive value of gonioscopy is relatively poor in determining which susceptible eyes will develop overt angle closure, even when gonioscopy is performed by experienced clinicians. Provocative tests such as pharmacologic pupillary dilation and the darkroom prone-position test have been used to precipitate a limited form of angle closure and thus predict which patients might develop angle closure. However, provocative testing has not been validated in a prospective study and is rarely used.

The decision to treat an asymptomatic patient with narrow angles rests on an accurate assessment of the anterior chamber angle and the clinical judgment of the ophthalmologist. Any patient with narrow angles should be advised of the symptoms of angle closure, the need for immediate ophthalmologic attention if symptoms occur, and the value of long-term periodic follow-up. An iridotomy is not necessary in all patients with a borderline narrow angle. A laser iridotomy should be considered in patients who have a narrow angle with documented appositional (ie, transient and intermittent) closure, PAS, increased segmental trabecular meshwork pigmentation, a history of previous angle closure, or other risk factors for angle closure (ACD <2.0 mm, strong family history). The status of the lens and the benefit of cataract surgery should also be considered in the decision.

A variety of factors that cause pupillary dilation—various drugs, pain, emotional upset, and fright, among others—may induce angle closure. In predisposed eyes with shallow anterior chambers, either mydriatic or miotic agents can precipitate acute angle closure (see the following subsection). Mydriatic agents include not only dilating drops but also systemic medications with sympathomimetic or anticholinergic activity that may cause pupillary dilation. The effect of miotics is to pull the peripheral iris away from the anterior chamber angle. However, strong miotics may also cause the zonular fibers of the lens to relax, allowing the lens–iris interface to move forward. Furthermore, their use results in greater iris–lens contact, thus potentially increasing pupillary block. For these reasons, miotics, especially the cholinesterase inhibitors, may induce or worsen angle closure. Gonioscopy should be repeated soon after miotic drugs are administered to patients with narrow angles.

Because of their potential for precipitating angle closure in susceptible individuals, a number of systemic medications that possess adrenergic (sympathomimetic) or anticholinergic (parasympatholytic) activity carry warnings against use by patients with glaucoma; these include allergy and cold medications, antidepressants, and some urological drugs. Although systemic administration generally does not raise intraocular drug levels to the same degree as topical administration, even slight mydriasis in a patient with a critically narrow angle can induce angle closure. When such drugs are administered to patients with potentially occludable angles, the ophthalmologist should inform the patient of the risk and consider performing iridotomy.

Foster PJ, Devereux JG, Alsbirk PH, et al. Detection of gonioscopically occludable angles and primary angle closure glaucoma by estimation of limbal chamber depth in Asians: modified grading scheme. *Br J Ophthalmol.* 2000;84(2):186–192.

Acute Primary Angle Closure

In acute primary angle closure (PAC), IOP rises rapidly as a result of relatively sudden blockage of the trabecular meshwork by the iris. Acute PAC is typically manifested by ocular pain, headache, blurred vision, and rainbow-colored halos around lights. Acute systemic distress may result in nausea and vomiting. The rise in IOP to relatively high levels causes corneal epithelial edema, which is responsible for the visual symptoms. Signs of acute angle closure include

- high IOP
- mid-dilated, sluggish, and irregularly shaped pupil
- corneal epithelial edema
- congested episcleral and conjunctival blood vessels
- shallow peripheral anterior chamber
- mild amount of aqueous flare and cells

Definitive diagnosis depends on the gonioscopic verification of angle closure. Gonioscopy should be possible in almost all cases of acute angle closure, although clearing of corneal edema with topical IOP-lowering therapy, topical glycerin, or paracentesis may be necessary to enable visualization of the angle. Dynamic gonioscopy, with indentation of the central cornea, may help the clinician determine whether the iris–trabecular meshwork blockage is reversible (appositional closure) or irreversible (synechial closure), and it may also be therapeutic in breaking the attack of acute angle closure. Gonioscopy of the fellow eye in a patient with PAC usually reveals a narrow, occludable angle. The presence of a deep angle in the fellow eye should prompt the clinician to search for secondary causes of elevated IOP, such as a posterior segment mass, zonular insufficiency, or the iridocorneal endothelial (ICE) syndrome. When performing gonioscopy, the clinician should observe the effect that the examination light has on the angle recess. For example, the pupillary constriction stimulated by the slit-lamp beam itself may open the angle and the narrow recess may go unrecognized (Fig 5-1).

During an acute attack, the IOP may be high enough to cause glaucomatous optic nerve damage, ischemic nerve damage, and/or retinal vascular occlusion. PAS can form rapidly, and IOP-induced ischemia may produce sector atrophy of the iris, releasing

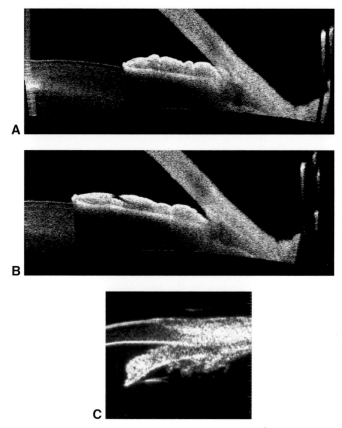

Figure 5-1 Ultrasound biomicroscopy (UBM) of a narrow angle. **A,** Angle closure is evident when the angle is imaged with lights off. **B,** The same angle is much more open when it is imaged with lights on. **C,** UBM of a narrow angle due to plateau iris. *(Parts A and B courtesy of Yaniv Barkana, MD; part C courtesy of Wallace L. M. Alward, MD.)*

pigment. This causes pigmentary dusting of the iris surface and corneal endothelium. Iris ischemia, specifically of the iris sphincter muscle, may cause the pupil to become permanently fixed and dilated. *Glaukomflecken,* characteristic small anterior subcapsular lens opacities, may also develop as a result of necrosis. These findings are helpful in the detection of previous episodes of acute PAC.

The definitive treatment of acute angle closure associated with pupillary block is usually laser iridotomy (discussed later), but mild attacks may be broken by cholinergic agents (pilocarpine 1%–2%), which induce miosis that pulls the peripheral iris away from the trabecular meshwork. However, these agents may worsen some types of angle closure without pupillary block. Stronger miotics should be avoided, as they may increase the vascular congestion of the iris or rotate the lens–iris interface more anteriorly, increasing the pupillary block. Moreover, when the IOP is markedly elevated (eg, >40–50 mm Hg), the pupillary sphincter may be ischemic and unresponsive to miotic agents alone. In this case, the patient should be treated with other topical agents, including β-adrenergic antagonists, α₂-adrenergic agonists, or prostaglandin analogues; or with topical, oral, or intravenous carbonic anhydrase inhibitors. A hyperosmotic agent may be administered orally or intravenously or a paracentesis can be performed with a 30-gauge needle or sharp blade. Globe compression over the central cornea, dynamic gonioscopy, and careful paracentesis with a sharp blade are all techniques to acutely lower the IOP in order to clear the corneal edema and allow laser iridotomy. Care should be taken, as the lens or iris can be easily injured when these techniques are employed. Argon laser peripheral iridoplasty may also help relieve acute attacks. Nonselective adrenergic agonists or medications with significant α_1-adrenergic activity (apraclonidine) should be avoided to prevent further pupillary dilation and iris ischemia.

In most cases of PAC, the fellow eye shares the anatomical predisposition for increased pupillary block and is at high risk of developing acute angle closure, especially if the inciting mechanism included a systemic sympathomimetic agent such as a nasal decongestant or an anticholinergic agent. In addition, the pain and emotional upset resulting from the involvement of the first eye may increase sympathetic flow to the fellow eye, resulting in pupillary dilation. It is recommended that a peripheral iridotomy be performed in the fellow eye if a similar angle configuration is present.

Laser iridotomy is the treatment of choice for acute PAC due to pupillary block. Much less commonly, a surgical iridectomy is used; these procedures are discussed in Chapter 8. Lensectomy is also a viable treatment option, although laser iridotomy may be more easily accomplished in the acute setting, especially if the eye is inflamed. Once an iridotomy has been performed, the pupillary block is relieved and the pressure gradient between the posterior and anterior chambers is normalized, which in most cases allows the iris to fall away from the trabecular meshwork. As a result, the anterior chamber deepens and the angle opens. If a laser iridotomy cannot be performed, the acute attack may be broken by flattening the peripheral iris with laser iridoplasty, relieving the pupillary block with laser pupilloplasty, or performing an iridectomy or lensectomy with goniosynechialysis. In such cases, a peripheral iridotomy/iridectomy should be performed, if not already done, once the attack is broken and the cornea is of adequate clarity. Following resolution of the acute attack, it is important to reevaluate the angle by gonioscopy to assess the degree of residual synechial angle closure and to confirm the reopening of at least part of the angle.

Improved IOP does not necessarily mean that the angle has opened. Because of ciliary body ischemia and reduced aqueous production, the IOP may remain low for weeks following acute angle closure. Thus, IOP may be a poor indicator of angle function or anatomy. A second gonioscopy or serial gonioscopy is therefore essential for follow-up of the patient to be certain that the angle has adequately opened.

Lam DS, Leung DY, Tham CC, et al. Randomized trial of early phacoemulsification versus peripheral iridotomy to prevent intraocular pressure rise after acute primary angle closure. *Ophthalmology.* 2008;115(7):1134–1140.

Subacute or Intermittent Angle Closure

Subacute or intermittent angle closure is a condition characterized by episodes of blurred vision, halos, and mild pain caused by elevated IOP. Vague symptoms of pain or headache not associated with visual symptoms have a low specificity for angle closure. The visual symptoms resolve spontaneously, especially during sleep-induced miosis, and the IOP is usually normal between episodes, which occur periodically over days, months, or years.

These episodes are often confused with headaches or migraines, so a careful history is required. The correct diagnosis can be made only with a high index of suspicion and gonioscopy. The typical history and the gonioscopic appearance of a narrow angle with or without PAS help establish the diagnosis. Such episodes may occur in the absence of symptoms as well, and are identified by elevated IOP or the presence of PAS in the setting of a narrow angle.

Laser iridotomy is the treatment of choice in subacute angle closure unless significant lens opacity is present, in which case lensectomy is typically curative. This condition can progress to chronic angle closure or to an acute attack that does not resolve spontaneously. With improvements in phacoemulsification, especially in terms of anterior chamber stabilization and fluidic control, primary lensectomy is increasingly recognized as an effective treatment for this disorder. In cases of significant synechial closure, goniosynechialysis may be performed in conjunction with lensectomy to help open the angle and improve trabecular outflow. Such treatment is more definitive than iridotomy but also introduces the additional risks inherent in intraocular surgery.

Chronic Angle Closure

Chronic angle closure may develop after acute angle closure in which synechial closure persists. It may also develop when the angle closes gradually and IOP rises slowly as angle function progressively becomes compromised. The latter form of chronic angle closure, in which there is gradual asymptomatic angle closure, is the most common presentation of angle closure. Because of the asymptomatic nature of this condition, vision loss may be the presenting concern. Accordingly, this disease tends to be diagnosed in its later stages. It is a major cause of blindness in Asia. Chronic PAC is often referred to as *creeping angle closure* because of the slow formation of PAS, which advance circumferentially. The cause of the phenomenon is uncertain, but evidence suggests that multiple mechanisms are involved, including pupillary block, abnormalities in iris thickness and position, and plateau iris configuration.

In chronic PAC, permanent PAS are present, as determined by indentation gonioscopy. The clinical course resembles that of open-angle glaucoma in its lack of symptoms, initial modest elevation of IOP, progressive glaucomatous optic nerve damage, and characteristic visual field loss. Over time, however, IOP can rise precipitously and become more difficult to control. The diagnosis of chronic PAC is frequently overlooked, and this condition is commonly confused with chronic open-angle glaucoma. As previously mentioned, gonioscopic examination of all glaucoma patients is important for accurate diagnosis.

Even if miotics and other agents lower the IOP, an iridotomy is necessary to relieve the pupillary block component and reduce the potential for further synechial angle closure. Without an iridotomy, closure of the angle usually progresses and makes the subsequent glaucoma more difficult to control. Even with a patent peripheral iridotomy, progressive angle closure can occur, and repeated periodic gonioscopy is imperative. An iridotomy with or without long-term use of ocular hypotensive medication controls the disease in most patients with chronic PAC. Others may require iridoplasty or lensectomy with or without goniosynechialysis. If these measures fail to lower the IOP, subsequent filtering surgery may be necessary.

Ritch R, Lowe RF. Angle closure glaucoma: clinical types. In: Ritch R, Shields MB, Krupin T, eds. *The Glaucomas*. 2nd ed. St Louis: Mosby; 1996:821–840.

Ritch R, Lowe RF. Angle closure glaucoma: mechanisms and epidemiology. In: Ritch R, Shields MB, Krupin T, eds. *The Glaucomas*. 2nd ed. St Louis: Mosby; 1996:801–819.

Plateau Iris Syndrome

Plateau iris refers to an atypical configuration of the anterior chamber angle that may result in acute or chronic PAC. Angle closure in plateau iris is most often caused by anteriorly positioned ciliary processes that critically narrow the anterior chamber recess by pushing the peripheral iris forward. Evidence suggests that plateau iris configuration may result from a more anterior junction of the iris dilator muscle and the ciliary epithelium, which causes the iris root to be more articulated. A component of pupillary block is often present. The angle may be further compromised following dilation of the pupil as the peripheral iris bunches up and obstructs the trabecular meshwork. Plateau iris may be suspected if the central anterior chamber appears to be of normal depth and the iris plane appears flat for an eye with angle closure. This suspicion can be confirmed by the presence of the "double-hump" sign on gonioscopy or ultrasound biomicroscopy (Fig 5-2). The condition will be missed if the examiner relies solely on the slit-lamp examination or the Van Herick method of angle examination.

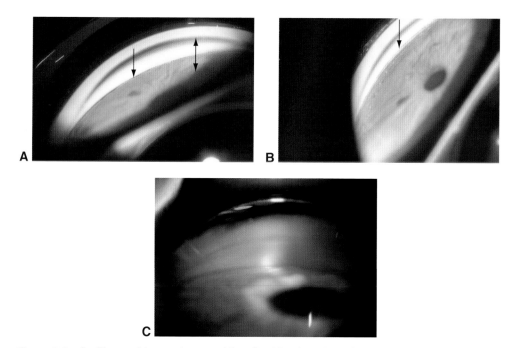

Figure 5-2 **A,** Plateau iris syndrome with a flat iris plane but shallow angle recess *(arrow)*. Note that the midperipheral angle appears deeper *(double arrow)* than the narrow angles associated with pupillary block. **B,** Plateau iris syndrome following laser peripheral iridoplasty, with a much deeper angle recess *(arrow)*. **C,** Plateau iris syndrome showing the classic "double-hump" sign. *(Parts A and B courtesy of M. Roy Wilson, MD; part C courtesy of Wallace L. M. Alward, MD.)*

The initial management of plateau iris includes either laser iridotomy to remove any component of pupillary block or lensectomy if cataract is present. Eyes with plateau iris syndrome remain predisposed to angle closure despite a patent iridotomy, as a result of the peripheral iris anatomy. Thus, careful assessment of the angle following iridotomy or lensectomy is necessary to determine whether additional treatment to further deepen the angle is required. PAS formation has been reported to begin at the Schwalbe line and then to extend in a posterior direction over the trabecular meshwork, scleral spur, and angle recess. The reverse is seen in pupillary block–induced angle closure, in which PAS form in the posterior to anterior direction. Patients with plateau iris syndrome may be treated with long-term miotic therapy. However, argon laser peripheral iridoplasty may be more useful in individuals with this condition to flatten and thin the peripheral iris (see Fig 5-2). Repeated gonioscopy at regular intervals is necessary because of the risk of chronic angle closure despite measures to deepen the angle recess.

Li Y, Wang YE, Huang G, et al. Prevalence and characteristics of plateau iris configuration among American Caucasian, American Chinese and mainland Chinese subjects. *Br J Ophthalmol.* 2014;98(4):474–478.

Pavlin CJ, Foster FS. Plateau iris syndrome: changes in angle opening associated with dark, light, and pilocarpine administration. *Am J Ophthalmol.* 1999;128(3): 288–291.

Secondary Angle Closure With Pupillary Block

Lens-Induced Angle Closure

Phacomorphic glaucoma

The mechanism of phacomorphic glaucoma is typically multifactorial. However, by definition, a significant component of the pathologic angle narrowing is related to the acquired mass effect of the cataractous lens itself. As with PAC, pupillary block often plays an important role in this condition. Phacomorphic narrowing of the angle generally occurs slowly with formation of the cataract. However, in some cases, the onset may be acute and rapid, precipitated by marked lens swelling (intumescence) as a result of cataract formation and the development of pupillary block in an eye that is otherwise not anatomically predisposed to closure (Figs 5-3, 5-4). Distinguishing between PAC and phacomorphic angle closure is not always straightforward and may not be necessary, as the treatment of both conditions is similar. However, the ACD, gonioscopic appearance, and degree of cataract differ between eyes with PAC and those with phacomorphic angle closure, and these differences can help the clinician determine the etiology. (See also BCSC Section 11, *Lens and Cataract.*) A laser iridotomy followed by cataract extraction in a quiet eye is the preferred treatment. In many cases, the iridotomy is unnecessary, as cataract surgery is the definitive treatment in eyes that have the potential for improved vision. Cholinergic agents have a minimal role in the treatment of this condition because they may further narrow the angle and worsen the vision in the presence of cataract. Further, the miotic pupil makes subsequent cataract surgery more challenging.

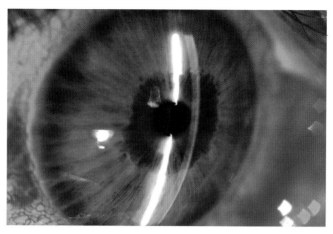

Figure 5-3 Phacomorphic glaucoma. Lens intumescence precipitates pupillary block and secondary angle closure in an eye not anatomically predisposed to angle closure. *(Courtesy of Wallace L. M. Alward, MD. From the Iowa Glaucoma Curriculum [curriculum.iowaglaucoma.org]. © The University of Iowa.)*

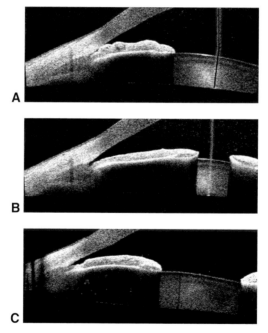

Figure 5-4 Phacomorphic glaucoma. **A,** In this example, the angle remains narrow despite a patent iridotomy. **B,** In bright light, the angle is transiently made deeper by pupil constriction. **C,** In this case, a more long-term solution is provided by thinning the peripheral iris with argon laser iridoplasty. Lensectomy is also a viable treatment strategy. *(Courtesy of Yaniv Barkana, MD.)*

Ectopia lentis

Ectopia lentis is defined as displacement of the lens from its normal anatomical position (Fig 5-5). With forward displacement, pupillary block may occur, resulting in iris bombé, shallowing of the anterior chamber angle, and secondary angle closure. The treatment of choice is performance of 2 laser iridotomies 180° apart. This relieves the pupillary block

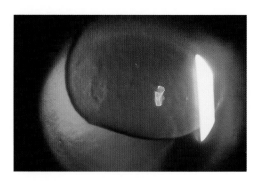

Figure 5-5 Ectopia lentis: dislocation of the lens into the anterior chamber through a dilated pupil. *(Courtesy of Ron Gross, MD.)*

Table 5-3 **Common Causes of Ectopia Lentis**
Pseudoexfoliation syndrome
Trauma
Marfan syndrome
Homocystinuria
Microspherophakia
Weill-Marchesani syndrome
Ehlers-Danlos syndrome
Sulfite oxidase deficiency

---

and is a temporizing measure until more definitive lensectomy, if indicated to improve visual function, can be performed. Lens extraction is usually indicated to restore vision and to reduce the risk of recurrent pupillary block and chronic angle closure development. See Table 5-3 for a list of conditions that can cause ectopia lentis.

Microspherophakia, a congenital disorder in which the lens has a spherical or globular shape, may cause ectopia lentis and subsequent pupillary block and PAC (Fig 5-6). Treatment with cycloplegia may tighten the zonule, flatten the lens, and pull it posteriorly, breaking the pupillary block. Miotics may make the condition worse by increasing the pupillary block and by rotating the ciliary body forward, loosening the zonule and allowing the lens to become more globular. Microspherophakia is often familial and may occur as an isolated condition or as part of either Weill-Marchesani or Marfan syndrome. The most common form of acquired zonular insufficiency and crystalline lens subluxation occurs in the pseudoexfoliation syndrome (Fig 5-7).

Aphakic or pseudophakic angle-closure glaucoma

Pupillary block may occur in *aphakic* and *pseudophakic* eyes. An intact vitreous face can block the pupil and/or an iridotomy site in aphakic or pseudophakic eyes or in a phakic eye with a dislocated lens. Generally, the anterior chamber shallows and the iris shows considerable bombé configuration. Treatment with mydriatic and cycloplegic agents may restore the aqueous flow through the pupil but may also make performing a laser iridotomy difficult initially. Topical β-adrenergic antagonists, α_2-adrenergic agonists, carbonic anhydrase inhibitors, and hyperosmotic agents can be effective in reducing IOP prior to performing an iridotomy. One or more laser iridotomies may be required.

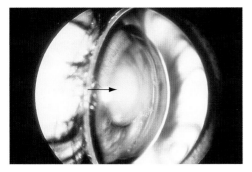

Figure 5-6 Ectopia lentis due to microsphe-rophakia. The lens *(arrow)* is trapped anteri-orly by the pupil, resulting in iris bombé and a dramatic shallowing of the anterior chamber. *(Courtesy of G. L. Spaeth, MD.)*

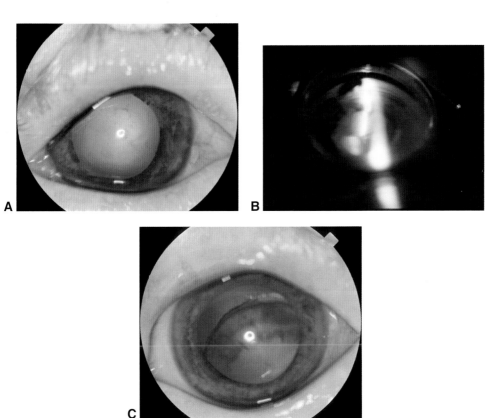

Figure 5-7 Pseudoexfoliation syndrome is a common cause of subluxation of the crystalline lens. **A,** Right eye of a patient with complete dislocation of the lens. **B,** Gonioscopic view of the same eye reveals that the dislocated lens is in the inferior vitreous cavity. **C,** Left eye (same patient) showing subluxation of the lens. *(Courtesy of Thomas W. Samuelson, MD.)*

Pupillary block may also occur with *anterior chamber intraocular lenses.* Pupillary block develops with apposition of the iris, vitreous face, and/or lens optic. The lens hap-tic or vitreous may obstruct the iridectomy site or the pupil, and the peripheral iris bows forward around the anterior chamber intraocular lens to occlude the angle. The central chamber remains deep relative to the peripheral chamber in this instance, because the lens haptic and optic prevent the central portions of the iris and vitreous face from moving forward. Laser iridotomies, often multiple, are required to relieve the block.

In addition, pupillary block may occur following posterior capsulotomy when vitreous obstructs the pupil. A condition referred to as *capsular block* may also be seen, whereby retained viscoelastic or fluid in the capsular bag pushes a posterior chamber intraocular lens anteriorly, which may narrow the angle.

Secondary Angle Closure Without Pupillary Block

A number of disorders can lead to secondary angle closure without pupillary block. This form of secondary angle closure may occur through 1 of 2 mechanisms:

- contraction of an inflammatory, hemorrhagic, or vascular membrane, band, or exudate in the angle, leading to PAS formation
- forward displacement of the lens–iris interface, often accompanied by swelling and anterior rotation of the ciliary body

Neovascular Glaucoma

This common, severe type of secondary angle closure is caused by a variety of disorders characterized by retinal or ocular ischemia or ocular inflammation (Table 5-4). The most common causes are diabetic retinopathy, central retinal vein occlusion (CRVO), branch retinal vein occlusion (BRVO), and ocular ischemic syndrome. The disease is characterized by fine arborizing blood vessels on the surface of the iris, pupillary margin, and trabecular meshwork, which are accompanied by a fibrous membrane.

Table 5-4 Disorders Predisposing to Neovascularization of the Iris and Angle

Systemic vascular disease	**Other ocular disease**
Carotid occlusive disease*	Chronic uveitis
Carotid artery ligation	Chronic retinal detachment
Carotid-cavernous fistula	Endophthalmitis
Giant cell arteritis	Stickler syndrome
Takayasu (pulseless) disease	Retinoschisis
Ocular vascular disease	**Intraocular tumors**
Diabetic retinopathy*	Uveal melanoma
Central retinal vein occlusion*	Metastatic carcinoma
Central retinal artery occlusion	Retinoblastoma
Branch retinal vein occlusion	Lymphoma
Sickle cell retinopathy	Reticulum cell sarcoma
Coats disease	**Ocular therapy**
Eales disease	Radiation therapy
Retinopathy of prematurity	**Trauma**
Persistent fetal vasculature	
Syphilitic vasculitis	
Anterior segment ischemia	

---

*Most common causes.

Neovascularization of the anterior segment usually presents in a classic pattern, which starts with fine vascular tufts at the pupillary margin (Fig 5-8). As these vessels grow, they extend radially over the iris. Unlike dilated stromal vessels, these vessels are delicate and lacey and do not adhere to the normal anterior segment vasculature. Further, when they involve the angle, they cross the ciliary body face and scleral spur as fine single vessels that then branch as they reach and involve the trabecular meshwork (see Chapter 3, Fig 3-6). Often the trabecular meshwork takes on a reddish coloration. With contraction of the fibrovascular membrane, PAS develop and coalesce, gradually closing the angle (Fig 5-9). While the fibrovascular membrane, like ICE syndrome, can cause ectropion uveae, it

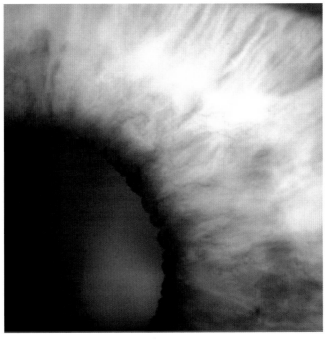

Figure 5-8 The initial presentation of iris neovascularization is usually small vascular tufts at the pupillary margin. *(Courtesy of Wallace L. M. Alward, MD. From the Iowa Glaucoma Curriculum [curriculum .iowaglaucoma.org]. © The University of Iowa.)*

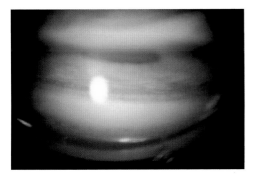

Figure 5-9 Iris neovascularization. With progressive angle involvement, PAS develop with contraction of the fibrovascular membrane, resulting in secondary neovascular glaucoma. *(Courtesy of Wallace L. M. Alward, MD. From the Iowa Glaucoma Curriculum [curriculum.iowa glaucoma.org]. © The University of Iowa.)*

typically does not grow over healthy corneal endothelium (Figs 5-10, 5-11). Thus, the PAS end at the Schwalbe line, distinguishing this condition from ICE syndrome.

Clinically, patients often present with an acute or subacute glaucoma associated with reduced vision, ocular pain, conjunctival hyperemia, microcystic corneal edema, and high IOP. While performing gonioscopy in patients with possible neovascularization, the clinician may find it helpful to use a bright slit-lamp beam of light and high magnification in order to best visualize these fine vessels.

In rare instances, anterior segment neovascularization may occur without demonstrable retinal ischemia, as in Fuchs heterochromic uveitis and other types of uveitis, pseudoexfoliation syndrome, or isolated iris melanomas. When an ocular cause cannot be found, carotid artery occlusive disease should be considered. In establishing a correct diagnosis, the clinician should distinguish dilated iris vessels associated with inflammation from newly formed abnormal blood vessels.

Because the prognosis for neovascular glaucoma is poor, prevention and early diagnosis are essential. In CRVO, angle neovascularization develops without iris neovascularization

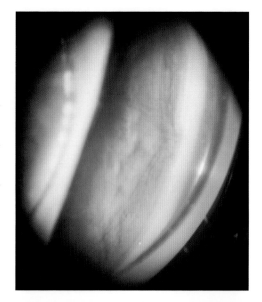

Figure 5-10 With end-stage neovascular glaucoma, total angle closure occurs, obscuring the iris neovascularization. The PAS end at the Schwalbe line because the fibrovascular membrane does not grow over healthy corneal endothelium. *(Courtesy of Wallace L. M. Alward, MD. From the Iowa Glaucoma Curriculum [curriculum.iowaglaucoma.org]. © The University of Iowa.)*

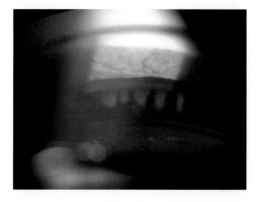

Figure 5-11 With vessel growth, iris neovascularization extends from the pupillary margin radially toward the anterior chamber angle. *(Courtesy of Wallace L. M. Alward, MD. From the Iowa Glaucoma Curriculum [curriculum.iowaglaucoma.org]. © The University of Iowa.)*

in approximately 10% of patients. Thus, gonioscopy is vital for early diagnosis. Since the most common cause of iris neovascularization is ischemic retinopathy, the definitive treatment when the ocular media are clear is panretinal photocoagulation. However, anti–vascular endothelial growth factor (anti-VEGF) therapy (eg, bevacizumab) can be used to acutely reduce the neovascular stimulus. The resulting decrease in neovascularization after panretinal photocoagulation may lower or normalize the IOP, depending on the extent of synechial closure. Even in the presence of total synechial angle closure, panretinal photocoagulation may improve the success rate of subsequent glaucoma surgery by eliminating the angiogenic stimulus and may decrease the risk of hemorrhage at the time of surgery. More recently, anti-VEGF agents have been successfully employed to promote regression of the neovascular tissue prior to filtering surgery (Fig 5-12) and improve outcome.

Medical management of neovascular glaucoma yields variable success and is only a temporizing measure until more definitive incisional or laser surgery is undertaken. Topical β-adrenergic antagonists, α_2-adrenergic agonists, carbonic anhydrase inhibitors, cycloplegics, and corticosteroids may be useful in reducing IOP and decreasing inflammation either as a long-term remedy or prior to filtering surgery. Filtering surgery or tube shunt implantation has a better chance of success once the neovascularization has regressed after panretinal photocoagulation or anti-VEGF therapy. A variety of tube shunts have also been successfully implanted to control the IOP in neovascular glaucoma and, in many cases, tube shunt implantation is the surgical procedure of choice. If these therapies fail or if the eye has poor visual potential, either endoscopic or transscleral cyclophotocoagulation can be considered as an alternative to filtering surgery or tube shunt implantation. See Chapter 8 for discussion of these procedures.

Iliev ME, Domig D, Wolf-Schnurrbursch U, Wolf S, Sarra GM. Intravitreal bevacizumab (Avastin) in the treatment of neovascular glaucoma. *Am J Ophthalmol.* 2006;142(6): 1054–1056.

Jonas JB, Spandau UH, Schlichtenbrede F. Intravitreal bevacizumab for filtering surgery. *Ophthalmic Res.* 2007;39(2):121–122.

Sivak-Callcott JA, O'Day DM, Gass JD, Tsai JC. Evidence-based recommendations for the diagnosis and treatment of neovascular glaucoma. *Ophthalmology.* 2001;108(10): 1767–1776.

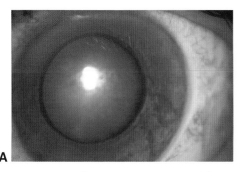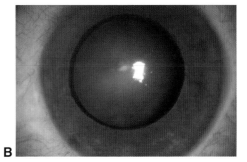

Figure 5-12   **A,** Slit-lamp photograph of florid iris neovascularization taken 15 minutes before injection of bevacizumab. **B,** Regression of iris neovascularization 4 days after treatment with bevacizumab. *(Courtesy of Nicholas P. Bell, MD.)*

Iridocorneal Endothelial Syndrome

Iridocorneal endothelial (ICE) syndrome is a group of disorders characterized by abnormal corneal endothelium that causes variable degrees of iris atrophy, secondary angle closure, and corneal edema. BCSC Section 8, *External Disease and Cornea,* discusses the corneal aspects of ICE syndrome. Three clinical variants have been described: Chandler syndrome, essential (progressive) iris atrophy, and Cogan-Reese syndrome (iris nevus). Chandler syndrome is the most common of the clinical variants, accounting for approximately 50% of the cases of ICE syndrome.

ICE syndrome is clinically unilateral, presents between 20 and 50 years of age, and occurs more often in women. No consistent association has been found with another ocular or systemic disease, and familial cases are very rare. Patients typically present with elevated IOP, decreased vision due to corneal edema, secondary chronic ACG, or an abnormal iris appearance. In each of the 3 clinical variants, the abnormal corneal endothelium takes on a "beaten bronze" appearance, similar to the cornea guttae seen in Fuchs corneal endothelial dystrophy. Microcystic corneal edema may be present without elevated IOP, especially in Chandler syndrome. The unaffected eye may have subclinical irregularities of the corneal endothelium without other manifestations of the disease.

High PAS are characteristic of ICE syndrome (Fig 5-13), and these often extend anterior to the Schwalbe line. The degree of angle closure does not always correlate to the elevation in IOP, because some angles may be functionally closed by the endothelial membrane without overt formation of synechiae.

Various degrees of iris atrophy and corneal changes distinguish the specific clinical entities. The *essential iris atrophy variant* of ICE syndrome is characterized by severe progressive iris atrophy resulting in heterochromia, corectopia, ectropion uveae, iris stromal and pigment epithelial atrophy, and hole formation (Fig 5-14). In *Chandler syndrome,* minimal iris atrophy and corectopia occur, and the corneal and angle findings predominate (Fig 5-15). The iris atrophy also tends to be less severe in *Cogan-Reese syndrome,* a condition distinguished by tan pedunculated nodules or diffuse pigmented lesions on the anterior iris surface.

Glaucoma develops in approximately 50% of patients with ICE syndrome and may be more severe in essential iris atrophy and Cogan-Reese syndrome. In ICE, the corneal endothelium migrates posterior to the Schwalbe line, onto the trabecular meshwork. Electron microscopy has shown the endothelium to vary in thickness, with areas of single

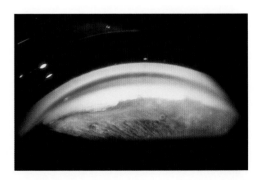

Figure 5-13 The classic high PAS of iridocorneal endothelial (ICE) syndrome. These PAS extend anterior to the Schwalbe line in this patient with essential iris atrophy. With angle closure, the secondary glaucoma develops. *(Courtesy of Steven T. Simmons, MD.)*

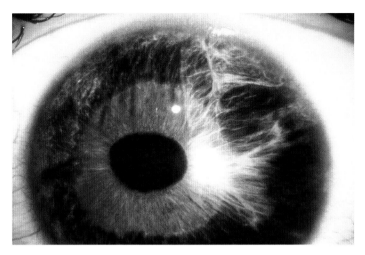

Figure 5-14 ICE syndrome. Clinical photograph showing corectopia and hole formation, typical findings in essential iris atrophy. *(Courtesy of Steven T. Simmons, MD.)*

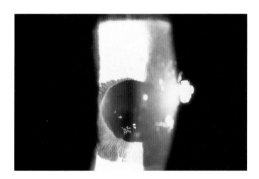

Figure 5-15 Clinical photograph showing ectropion uveae in a patient with Chandler syndrome. *(Courtesy of Steven T. Simmons, MD.)*

and multiple endothelial layers and surrounding collagenous and fibrillar tissue. Unlike with normal corneal endothelium, filopodial processes and cytoplasmic actin filaments are present, supporting the migratory nature of these cells. PAS are formed when this migratory endothelium and its surrounding collagenous, fibrillar tissue contract. A virus has been postulated as the etiology of ICE syndrome after lymphocytes were observed on the corneal endothelium of affected patients.

The diagnosis of ICE syndrome must always be considered in young to middle-aged patients who present with unilateral, secondary angle closure. It is particularly important to maintain a high index of suspicion for this condition, because it may mimic primary open-angle glaucoma when the iris and corneal features are subtle. Specular microscopy can confirm the diagnosis by demonstrating an asymmetric loss of endothelial cells and atypical endothelial cell morphology in the involved eye.

Therapy is directed toward the corneal edema and secondary glaucoma. Hypertonic saline solutions and medications to reduce the IOP, when elevated, can be effective in controlling the corneal edema. The ACG, when present, can be treated medically with aqueous suppressants and prostaglandin analogues. Miotics are often ineffective. When medical therapy fails, filtering surgery (trabeculectomy or a tube shunt) can be effective. Late failures have been reported with trabeculectomy secondary to endothelialization of the fistula. The fistula can be reopened in some cases with the Nd:YAG laser. Laser trabeculoplasty has no useful role in treating glaucoma related to ICE syndrome.

Tumors

Tumors in the posterior segment of the eye or anterior uveal cysts may cause a unilateral secondary angle closure. Primary choroidal melanomas, ocular metastases, and retinoblastoma are the most common tumors to cause secondary angle closure. The mechanism of the angle closure is determined by the size, location, and pathology of the tumor. Choroidal and retinal tumors tend to shift the lens–iris interface forward as the tumors enlarge, causing secondary angle closure. Breakdown of the blood–aqueous barrier and inflammation from tissue necrosis can result in posterior synechiae and PAS formation, further exacerbating other underlying mechanisms of angle closure. Anterior segment neovascularization often occurs with retinoblastomas, medulloepitheliomas, and choroidal melanomas, as well as following radiation treatment, resulting in neovascular glaucoma.

Inflammation

Secondary angle closure can occur as a result of ocular inflammation. Fibrin and increased aqueous proteins released due to the breakdown of the blood–aqueous barrier may predispose the eye to formation of posterior synechiae (Fig 5-16) and PAS. If left untreated, these posterior synechiae can result in a secluded pupil, iris bombé, and secondary angle closure (Fig 5-17).

Peripheral iris edema, organization of inflammatory debris in the angle, and bridging of the angle by large keratic precipitates (eg, as seen in sarcoidosis) occur with the ocular inflammation and may lead to formation of PAS. These PAS form most frequently in the inferior anterior chamber angle, unlike the PAS in PAC, which typically occur in the superior angle. The PAS are usually not uniform in shape or height, further distinguishing inflammatory disease from PAC (Fig 5-18). In rare instances, ischemia secondary to inflammation may cause rubeosis iridis and neovascular glaucoma.

Ocular inflammation can lead to the shallowing and closure of the anterior chamber angle by uveal effusion, resulting in anterior rotation of the ciliary body. Significant

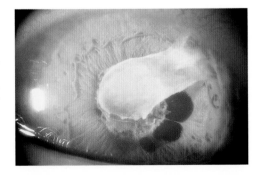

Figure 5-16 Inflammatory glaucoma in a patient with ankylosing spondylitis. A fibrinous anterior chamber reaction and posterior synechiae formation are evident. *(Courtesy of Steven T. Simmons, MD.)*

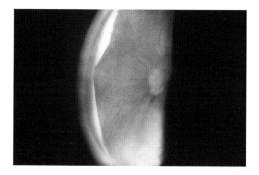

Figure 5-17 Clinical photograph showing inflammatory glaucoma. A secluded pupil is shown in a patient with long-standing uveitis with classic iris bombé and secondary angle closure. *(Courtesy of Steven T. Simmons, MD.)*

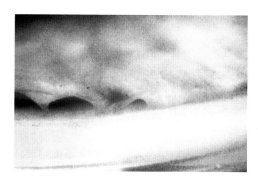

Figure 5-18 Inflammatory glaucoma. PAS in uveitis occur typically in the inferior anterior chamber angle and are nonuniform in height and shape, as shown in this photograph. *(Courtesy of Joseph Krug, MD.)*

posterior uveitis causing massive exudative retinal detachment or choroidal effusions may lead to ACG through forward displacement of the lens–iris interface. Treatment is primarily directed at the underlying cause of the uveitis. Aqueous suppressants and corticosteroids are the primary agents for reducing elevated IOP and preventing synechial angle closure.

Interstitial keratitis may be associated with open-angle glaucoma or angle closure. The angle closure may be caused by chronic inflammation and PAS formation or by multiple cysts of the iris pigment epithelium.

Sng CC, Barton K. Mechanism and management of angle closure in uveitis. *Curr Opin Ophthalmol.* 2015;26(2):121–127.

Malignant Glaucoma

Malignant glaucoma (also called aqueous misdirection or ciliary block glaucoma) is a rare but potentially devastating form of glaucoma that usually presents following ocular surgery in patients with a history of angle closure or PAS. It may also occur spontaneously in eyes with an open angle or following cataract surgery or various laser procedures. The disease presents with uniform flattening of both the central and peripheral anterior chamber (Fig 5-19), which is typically markedly asymmetrical to the anterior chamber of the fellow eye. This is in contrast to acute PAC, which presents with iris bombé and a shallow peripheral anterior chamber (Fig 5-20). Classically, the condition is thought to result from anterior rotation of the ciliary body and posterior misdirection of the aqueous, in association with a relative block to aqueous movement at the level of the lens equator, vitreous

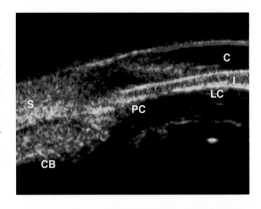

Figure 5-19 Malignant glaucoma viewed with UBM. Expansion of the vitreous pushes the lens and ciliary body forward, causing a uniform shallowing of the anterior chamber. The central portion of the anterior lens capsule (LC) is nearly in contact with the cornea (C). PC = posterior chamber; CB = ciliary body; I = iris; S = sclera. *(From Lundy DC. Ciliary block glaucoma.* Focal Points: Clinical Modules for Ophthalmologists. *San Francisco: American Academy of Ophthalmology; 1999, module 3. Courtesy of Jeffrey M. Liebmann, MD.)*

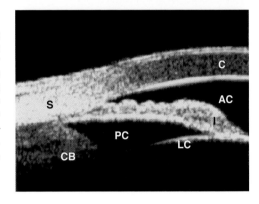

Figure 5-20 Acute angle closure viewed with UBM. Pupillary block leads to forward bowing of the peripheral iris. The peripheral chamber is shallow, whereas the central chamber is relatively deeper by comparison. C = cornea; AC = anterior chamber; PC = posterior chamber; LC = lens capsule; CB = ciliary body; I = iris; S = sclera. *(From Lundy DC. Ciliary block glaucoma.* Focal Points: Clinical Modules for Ophthalmologists. *San Francisco: American Academy of Ophthalmology; 1999, module 3. Courtesy of Jeffrey M. Liebmann, MD.)*

face, and ciliary processes. Some have proposed that PAC and malignant glaucoma may result from the simultaneous presence of several factors, including a small eye, a propensity for choroidal expansion, and reduced vitreous fluid conductivity.

Clinically, the anterior chamber is shallow or flat with anterior displacement of the lens, pseudophakos, or vitreous face. Optically clear "aqueous" zones may be seen in the vitreous, highlighting the underlying pathology. In the early postoperative setting, malignant glaucoma is often difficult to distinguish from choroidal effusion, pupillary block, or suprachoroidal hemorrhage. Often the level of IOP, time frame following surgery, patency of an iridotomy, or presence of a choroidal effusion or suprachoroidal hemorrhage helps the clinician make the appropriate diagnosis. In some cases, the clinical picture is difficult to interpret, and surgical intervention may be required in order to make the diagnosis.

Medical management includes the triad of intensive cycloplegic therapy; aggressive aqueous suppression with β-adrenergic antagonists, α_2-adrenergic agonists, and carbonic anhydrase inhibitors; and reducing the vitreous with hyperosmotic agents. Miotics can make malignant glaucoma worse and therefore should not be used. In aphakic and pseudophakic eyes, the anterior vitreous can be disrupted with the Nd:YAG laser. Argon laser photocoagulation of the ciliary processes reportedly has been helpful in treating this condition; this procedure may alter the adjacent vitreous face. In approximately half of patients, malignant glaucoma can be controlled with laser iridotomy and medical management; half of patients require surgical intervention alone. The definitive surgical treatment is pars plana vitrectomy with anterior hyaloido-zonulectomy combined with an anterior chamber deepening procedure. BCSC Section 12, *Retina and Vitreous,* discusses vitrectomy in detail.

Lundy DC. Ciliary block glaucoma. *Focal Points: Clinical Modules for Ophthalmologists.* San Francisco: American Academy of Ophthalmology; 1999, module 3.

Quigley HA, Friedman DS, Congdon NG. Possible mechanisms of primary angle-closure and malignant glaucoma. *J Glaucoma.* 2003;12(2):167–180.

Nonrhegmatogenous Retinal Detachment and Uveal Effusions

A nonrhegmatogenous retinal detachment occurs when subretinal fluid is present in the absence of a retinal break. A suprachoroidal effusion or hemorrhage refers to blood or fluid in the potential space between the choroid and the sclera. Retinoblastoma, Coats disease, metastatic carcinoma, choroidal melanoma, suprachoroidal hemorrhage, choroidal effusion/detachment, infections (eg, HIV), and subretinal neovascularization in age-related macular degeneration with extensive effusion or hemorrhage can cause nonrhegmatogenous retinal detachments. Suprachoroidal mass effect may result in secondary angle closure related to forward displacement of the lens–iris interface. See BCSC Section 12, *Retina and Vitreous,* for further discussion.

In a *rhegmatogenous retinal detachment,* the subretinal fluid can escape through the retinal tear and equalize the hydraulic pressure on both sides of the retina. In a nonrhegmatogenous retinal detachment, by contrast, the subretinal fluid accumulates and becomes a space-occupying lesion in the vitreous, which may progressively push the retina forward against the lens like a hydraulic press. The fluid or hemorrhage may accumulate rapidly, and as it pushes the retina forward to a retrolenticular position, it can in severe cases flatten the anterior chamber completely. The retina may be dramatically visible behind the lens on slit-lamp examination.

Epithelial and Fibrous Ingrowth

Epithelial and fibrous proliferations are rare surgical complications that can cause severe secondary glaucoma. Epithelial and fibrous ingrowth occurs when epithelium and/or connective tissue invades the anterior chamber through a defect in a wound site. Fortunately, improved surgical and wound closure techniques have greatly reduced the incidence of these entities. A common cause of corneal graft failure, fibrous ingrowth is more prevalent than epithelial ingrowth. Risk factors for development of these entities include prolonged inflammation, wound dehiscence, delayed wound closure, or a Descemet membrane tear. Epithelial ingrowth has also been reported following Descemet-stripping automated endothelial keratoplasty.

Epithelial ingrowth presents as a grayish, sheetlike growth on the trabecular meshwork, iris, ciliary body, and posterior surface of the cornea. It is often associated with vitreous incarceration, wound gape, ocular inflammation, hypotony secondary to choroidal effusions, and corneal edema (Figs 5-21, 5-22). The epithelial ingrowth consists of nonkeratinized stratified squamous epithelium with an avascular subepithelial connective tissue layer.

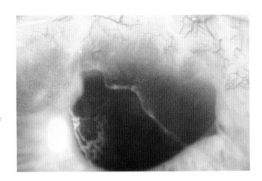

Figure 5-21 Epithelial ingrowth appears as a grayish, sheetlike growth on the endothelial surface of the cornea, usually originating from a surgical incision or traumatic wound. The epithelial ingrowth shown here originated from a cataract surgery incision. *(Courtesy of Steven T. Simmons, MD.)*

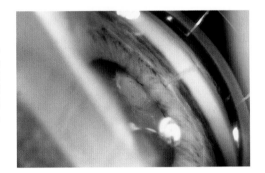

Figure 5-22 Epithelial ingrowth. The precipitating causes of epithelial ingrowth include vitreous incarceration in corneal and scleral wounds, as seen in this photograph, as well as wound gape, ocular inflammation, and hypotony secondary to choroidal effusions. *(Courtesy of Steven T. Simmons, MD.)*

The argon laser produces characteristic white burns on the epithelial membrane on the iris surface, which help to confirm the diagnosis of epithelial ingrowth and to determine the extent of involvement. If the diagnosis remains in question, a cytologic examination of an aqueous aspirate can be performed. Radical surgery is sometimes necessary to remove the intraocular epithelial membrane and the affected tissues and to repair the fistula, but the prognosis remains poor; thus the decision to intervene is made based on the extent of disease, the visual potential, the status of the fellow eye, and socio-medical circumstances relevant to the affected individual.

Fibrovascular tissue may also proliferate into an eye from a penetrating wound. Unlike epithelial proliferation, fibrous ingrowth progresses slowly and is often self-limited. Fibrous ingrowth appears as a thick, gray-white, vascular retrocorneal membrane with an irregular border. The ingrowth often involves the angle, resulting in PAS formation with destruction of the trabecular meshwork (Fig 5-23) and ectropion uveae. The resultant secondary angle closure is often difficult to control. Medication is the preferred treatment of the secondary glaucomas that present without a pupillary block mechanism, although surgical intervention may be required. See Chapters 7 and 8 for further discussion.

Trauma

Following ocular trauma, angle-closure glaucoma without pupillary block may develop from the formation of PAS associated with angle recession or from contusion, hyphema, and inflammation. See Chapter 4 for discussion of trauma.

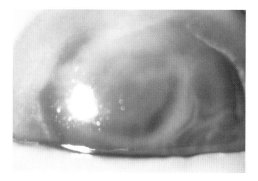

Figure 5-23 Fibrous ingrowth appears as a thick, grayish, vascular retrocorneal membrane that results in high PAS and destruction of the trabecular meshwork. *(Courtesy of Steven T. Simmons, MD.)*

Retinal Surgery and Retinal Vascular Disease

Used for surgical repair of retinal detachments, scleral buckles, especially the encircling bands, can produce shallowing of the anterior chamber angle and frank angle closure, often accompanied by choroidal effusion and anterior rotation of the ciliary body, causing a flattening of the peripheral iris with a relatively deep central anterior chamber. Usually, the anterior chamber deepens with opening of the anterior chamber angle over days to weeks with medical therapy consisting of cycloplegics, anti-inflammatory agents, β-adrenergic antagonists, carbonic anhydrase inhibitors, and hyperosmotic agents. If medical management is unsuccessful, argon laser iridoplasty, drainage of suprachoroidal fluid, or adjustment of the scleral buckle may be required. Iridectomy is usually of little benefit in this condition. The scleral buckle can impede venous drainage by compressing a vortex vein, elevating episcleral venous pressure and IOP. Such cases may respond only to moving the scleral buckle or releasing tension on the encircling band.

Following a pars plana vitrectomy, angle closure may result from the injection into the eye of air, long-acting gases such as sulfur hexafluoride and perfluorocarbons (perfluoropropane and perfluoroethane), or silicone oil. These substances are less dense than water and rise to the top of the eye. An iridotomy may be beneficial and should be located inferiorly to prevent obstruction of the iridotomy site by the gas or oil.

Eyes that have undergone complicated vitreoretinal surgery and have elevated IOP require individualized treatment plans. Treatment options include the following: removal of the silicone oil; release of the encircling element; removal of expansile gases; or primary glaucoma surgery, such as trabeculectomy, tube shunt implantation, or a cyclodestructive procedure.

Following panretinal photocoagulation, IOP may become elevated by an angle-closure mechanism. The ciliary body is thickened and rotated anteriorly, and often an anterior annular choroidal detachment occurs. Generally, this secondary glaucoma is self-limited, and therapy is directed at temporary medical management with cycloplegic agents, topical corticosteroids, and aqueous suppressants.

CRVO sometimes causes early shallowing of the angle, presumably because of swelling of the choroid and ciliary body. In rare cases, the angle becomes sufficiently compromised, leading to angle closure and elevated IOP. The chamber deepens and the angle closure resolves over 1 week to several weeks. Medical therapy for the elevated IOP, combined with administration of topical corticosteroids and cycloplegia, is usually preferred. However, if the contralateral eye of a patient with CRVO has a potentially occludable anterior chamber angle, the ophthalmologist must consider an underlying pupillary block mechanism and the possible need for bilateral iridotomy.

Nanophthalmos

A nanophthalmic eye is normal in shape but unusually small, with a shortened axial length (<20 mm), a small corneal diameter, and a relatively large lens for the volume of the eye. Thickened sclera may impede drainage from the vortex veins. These eyes are markedly hyperopic and highly susceptible to angle closure, which occurs at an earlier age than in PAC. Intraocular surgery is frequently complicated by choroidal effusion and nonrhegmatogenous retinal detachment. Choroidal effusion may occur spontaneously and may induce angle closure. Laser iridotomy, argon laser peripheral iridoplasty, and medical therapy are the safest ways to manage glaucoma in these patients. Surgery should be avoided if possible because of the high rate of surgical complications. When intraocular surgery is employed, prophylactic posterior sclerotomies may reduce the severity of intraoperative choroidal effusion. Additional treatment options include lensectomy for angles that remain compromised despite a patent iridotomy. In such cases, a limited core vitrectomy is sometimes necessary to provide adequate ACD for subsequent, safe lens removal. Many clinicians consider early lens extraction in patients with nanophthalmos to avoid the development of angle closure.

Persistent Fetal Vasculature

The contracting retrolental tissue seen in persistent fetal vasculature (PFV; formerly known as *persistent hyperplastic primary vitreous*) and in retinopathy of prematurity can cause progressive shallowing of the anterior chamber angle with subsequent angle closure. These conditions are discussed in more detail in BCSC Section 6, *Pediatric Ophthalmology and Strabismus,* and Section 12, *Retina and Vitreous.* In PFV, the onset of this complication usually occurs at 3–6 months of age during the cicatricial phase of the disease. However, the angle closure may occur later in childhood.

PFV is usually unilateral and often associated with microphthalmos and elongated ciliary processes. The contracture of the hyperplastic primary vitreous and swelling of a cataractous lens may result in subsequent angle closure.

Flat Anterior Chamber

A flat anterior chamber from any cause can result in the formation of PAS. Debate continues concerning how long a postoperative flat chamber should be treated conservatively before surgical intervention is undertaken. Hypotony in an eye with a postoperative flat chamber following cataract surgery or filtering surgery indicates a wound leak until proven otherwise. A Seidel test should be performed to locate the leak. Simple pressure patching or bandage contact lens application will often cause the leak to seal and the chamber to re-form. If the chamber does not re-form, the leak should be repaired surgically to prevent synechial closure of the angle or other complications of hypotony.

Some ophthalmologists repair the wound leak and re-form a flat chamber following cataract surgery within 24 hours. Others prefer observation in conjunction with corticosteroid therapy for several days to prevent formation of synechiae. Although iridocorneal contact is well tolerated, contact between the cornea and the hyaloid face or an IOL requires re-formation of the chamber without delay to minimize corneal endothelial damage. Early intervention should also be considered in the presence of corneal edema, excessive inflammation, or posterior synechiae formation.

Drug-Induced Secondary Angle-Closure Glaucoma

Topiramate, a sulfamate-substituted monosaccharide, is an oral medication prescribed in the treatment of epilepsy, depression, headaches, and idiopathic intracranial hypertension. In some patients, this medication may cause a syndrome characterized by acute myopic shift and acute bilateral angle closure. Patients with this syndrome experience sudden bilateral vision loss with acute myopia, bilateral ocular pain, and headache, usually within 1 month of starting topiramate. In addition to myopia, ocular findings of this syndrome include a uniformly shallow anterior chamber with anterior displacement of the iris and lens, microcystic corneal edema, elevated IOP (40–70 mm Hg), a closed anterior chamber angle, and a ciliochoroidal effusion/detachment (Fig 5-24). Other medications associated with uveal effusions with secondary angle closure include acetazolamide, methazolamide, and trimethoprim-sulfamethoxazole.

The bilateral nature of this form of angle closure should alert the clinician to the possibility of an idiosyncratic response to topiramate. Treatment of this syndrome involves immediate discontinuation of the medication and initiation of medical therapy to decrease the IOP, generally in the form of aqueous suppressants. In addition, systemic agents such as acetazolamide may be administered orally or intravenously. Aggressive cycloplegia may help deepen the anterior chamber and relieve the attack. The secondary angle closure usually resolves within 24–48 hours with medical treatment, and the

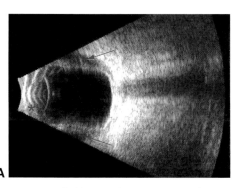
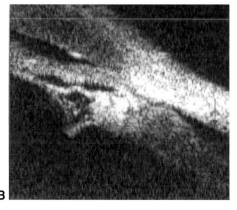

A   B

Figure 5-24 **A,** B-scan ultrasonogram of an eye with a very shallow anterior chamber *(asterisk)* and topiramate-induced angle-closure glaucoma. The choroidal effusion is clearly evident *(arrows)*. **B,** Ultrasonographic view of an extremely shallow anterior chamber and closed angle *(asterisk)*. The posterior choroidal effusion is clearly visible *(arrow)*. *(Courtesy of Jonathan Eisengart, MD.)*

myopia resolves within 1–2 weeks of discontinuing the topiramate. Because pupillary block is not an underlying mechanism of this syndrome, a peripheral iridotomy is not indicated. Other sulfonamides, such as acetazolamide, have been reported to cause a similar clinical syndrome.

Epstein DL, Allingham RR, Schuman JS, eds. *Chandler and Grant's Glaucoma.* 4th ed. Baltimore: Williams & Wilkins; 1997.

Lachkar Y, Bouassida W. Drug-induced acute angle closure glaucoma. *Curr Opin Ophthalmol.* 2007;18(2):129–133.

Ritch R, Shields MB, Krupin T, eds. *The Glaucomas.* 2nd ed. St Louis: Mosby; 1996.

Shields MB. *Textbook of Glaucoma.* 4th ed. Philadelphia: Williams & Wilkins; 2000.

Stamper RL, Lieberman MF, Drake MV, eds. *Becker-Shaffer's Diagnosis and Therapy of the Glaucomas.* 7th ed. St Louis: Mosby; 1999.

CHAPTER **6**

Glaucoma in Children and Adolescents

The glaucomas of childhood and adolescence (herein called pediatric glaucomas) are a heterogeneous group of disorders associated with elevated intraocular pressure (IOP) and optic nerve damage. Various presentations and etiologies characterize these rare glaucomas. Although pediatric glaucomas share many characteristics with adult-onset glaucomas, there are numerous management issues that are unique to the pediatric and adolescent populations.

See BCSC Section 6, *Pediatric Ophthalmology and Strabismus*, for additional discussion of many of the topics covered in this chapter.

Classification

Many systems have been used to classify the pediatric glaucomas. The World Glaucoma Association, for example, classifies them into primary and secondary glaucomas (see Table 22-1 in BCSC Section 6, *Pediatric Ophthalmology and Strabismus*). The classifications presented in Tables 6-1 and 6-2 in this book are based on anatomical anomalies, age of onset, inheritance, and associated systemic disorders. Most of these systems divide the glaucomas into primary and secondary glaucomas, although there is some overlap in this classification (eg, Sturge-Weber syndrome is both a primary and a secondary glaucoma). *Primary* pediatric glaucomas are developmental glaucomas with congenital anomalies of the filtration angle, and they can be subdivided as follows:

- primary congenital glaucoma (congenital open-angle glaucoma)
- juvenile open-angle glaucoma
- glaucoma associated with ocular developmental anomalies
- glaucoma associated with systemic diseases

Children with *primary congenital glaucoma (PCG)* present with enlarged and/or cloudy corneas, Haab striae, and elevated IOP—the classic features of PCG. PCG may present at birth or before 1 month of age (newborn PCG), within the first 2 years of life (infantile PCG), or after 2 years of age (late-diagnosed PCG). *Juvenile open-angle glaucoma* develops later in childhood or in early adulthood. Primary pediatric glaucomas are associated with abnormal development of the anterior segment, as in aniridia or Peters anomaly. In addition, primary pediatric glaucoma can be associated with a number of systemic diseases, including chromosomal disorders, connective tissue disorders (eg, Marfan and Stickler syndromes), and the phakomatoses.

Secondary pediatric glaucomas arise from multiple etiologies, including trauma, intraocular neoplasms, inflammation, lens-induced disorders, surgical interventions, angle closure, infection, neovascularization, corticosteroid use, or elevated episcleral venous pressure (see Table 6-2).

Table 6-1 Classification Scheme for Primary Pediatric Glaucomas

I. Primary congenital glaucomas
  A. Newborn glaucoma
  B. Infantile glaucoma
  C. Late-diagnosed glaucoma
II. Juvenile (open-angle) glaucoma
III. Associated with ocular abnormalities (anterior segment developmental abnormality)
  A. Axenfeld-Rieger syndrome
  B. Aniridia
  C. Congenital iris ectropion syndrome
  D. Iridotrabecular dysgenesis (iris hypoplasia)
  E. Peters anomaly
  F. Congenital microcornea with myopia
  G. Sclerocornea
  H. Congenital hereditary endothelial dystrophy
  I. Posterior polymorphous corneal dystrophy
  J. Megalocornea
IV. Associated with systemic abnormalities
  A. Chromosomal disorders
    1. Trisomy 13 (Patau syndrome)
    2. Trisomy 15
    3. Trisomy 18 (Edward syndrome)
    4. Trisomy 21 (Down syndrome)
    5. Turner syndrome (XO)
  B. Connective tissue abnormalities
    1. Marfan syndrome
    2. Stickler syndrome
    3. Others (see Table 6-2)
  C. Phakomatoses
    1. Sturge-Weber syndrome (isolated vs with central nervous system involvement)
    2. Neurofibromatosis 1
    3. Nevus of Ota (ocular melanosis)
    4. von Hippel–Lindau syndrome
  D. Other
    1. Hepatocerebrorenal syndrome (Zellweger syndrome)
    2. Kniest dysplasia
    3. Hallermann-Streiff syndrome
    4. Michel syndrome
    5. Nail-patella syndrome
    6. Oculodentodigital dysplasia
    7. Prader-Willi syndrome
    8. Rubinstein-Taybi syndrome
    9. Waardenburg syndrome
    10. Walker-Warburg syndrome
    11. Cutis marmorata telangiectasia congenita

Adapted from Yanovitch TL, Freedman SF. Pediatric glaucoma. *Focal Points: Clinical Modules for Ophthalmologists.* San Francisco: American Academy of Ophthalmology; 2012, module 3.

Table 6-2 Classification Scheme for Secondary Pediatric Glaucomas

I. Secondary to trauma
  A. Acute glaucoma
  B. Late-onset glaucoma with angle recession
  C. Arteriovenous fistula
II. Secondary to intraocular neoplasm
  A. Retinoblastoma
  B. Juvenile xanthogranuloma
  C. Leukemia
  D. Melanoma
  E. Melanocytoma
  F. Iris rhabdomyosarcoma
  G. Aggressive nevi of the iris
  H. Medulloepithelioma
III. Secondary to uveitis
  A. Open-angle glaucoma
  B. Angle-blockage glaucoma
    1. Synechial angle closure
    2. Iris bombé with pupillary block
    3. Trabecular endothelialization
IV. Lens-induced
  A. Subluxation or dislocation and pupillary block
    1. Marfan syndrome
    2. Homocystinuria
    3. Weill-Marchesani syndrome
    4. Ectopia lentis
    5. Hyperlysinemia
  B. Spherophakia with pupillary block
  C. Phacolytic glaucoma
V. After surgery for congenital cataract
  A. Lens tissue trabecular obstruction
  B. Pupillary block (angle closure)
  C. Chronic open-angle glaucoma associated with angle abnormalities
VI. Steroid-induced
VII. Secondary to rubeosis
  A. Retinoblastoma
  B. Coats disease
  C. Familial exudative vitreoretinopathy
  D. Medulloepithelioma
  E. Chronic retinal detachment
VIII. Secondary angle-closure glaucomas
  A. Retinopathy of prematurity
  B. Persistent fetal vasculature
  C. Microphthalmos
  D. Nanophthalmos
  E. Iris stromal cysts
  F. Ciliary body cysts
  G. Congenital pupillary iris–lens membrane
  H. Retinoblastoma
  I. Cystinosis
  J. Central retinal vein occlusion
  K. Topiramate-induced
IX. Malignant glaucoma

(Continued)

Table 6-2 *(continued)*
_____

  X. Glaucoma associated with increased episcleral venous pressure
     A. Sturge-Weber syndrome (isolated vs with central nervous system involvement)
     B. Cavernous or dural venous fistula
     C. Orbital disease
  XI. Secondary to maternal rubella
 XII. Secondary to intraocular infection
     A. Acute recurrent toxoplasmosis
     B. Acute herpetic iritis

Adapted from Yanovitch TL, Freedman SF. Pediatric glaucoma. *Focal Points: Clinical Modules for Ophthalmologists.* San Francisco: American Academy of Ophthalmology; 2012, module 3.

Yeung HH, Walton DS. Clinical classification of childhood glaucomas. *Arch Ophthalmol.* 2010;128(6):680–684.

Genetics

Most cases of PCG occur sporadically. A familial pattern of inheritance is seen in 10%–40% of cases, usually autosomal recessive with incomplete or variable penetrance. Linkage studies have identified 4 genetic loci of PCG—GLC3A, GLC3B, GLC3C, and GLC3D—but additional loci likely exist (see Chapter 1, Table 1-4). Two main genes associated with PCG have been identified:

- *CYP1B1* (cytochrome P450, family 1, subfamily B, polypeptide 1) within the GLC3A locus
- *LTBP2* (latent transforming growth factor beta-binding protein 2) within the GLC3C locus

Most cases of juvenile open-angle glaucoma have an autosomal dominant inheritance pattern, but sporadic cases occasionally occur. Juvenile open-angle glaucoma has been linked to mutations in the *TIGR* (trabecular meshwork inducible glucocorticoid response)/*MYOC* (myocilin) gene located at the GLC1A locus.

Some forms of primary pediatric glaucoma are associated with ocular abnormalities, including aniridia, Axenfeld-Rieger syndrome, and Peters anomaly. Aniridia results from mutations in the *PAX6* gene (paired box 6). Two-thirds of aniridia cases are autosomal dominant and one-third are sporadic. Axenfeld-Rieger syndrome has an autosomal dominant pattern of inheritance and presents with a variety of phenotypes. Mutations in the *PITX2* gene (paired-like homeodomain transcription factor 2), located at 4q25, and the *FOXC1* gene (forkhead box C1), located at 6p25, have been linked to this syndrome. The variable interaction between these 2 genes may underlie the diverse phenotypic expression associated with Axenfeld-Rieger syndrome. Peters anomaly has been linked to mutations in *PITX2, FOXC1, CYP1B1,* and *PAX6.*

Genetic testing should be considered for parents of pediatric glaucoma patients and for adults with onset of glaucoma in childhood or early adulthood.

Zhao Y, Sorenson CM, Sheibani N. Cytochrome P450 1B1 and primary congenital glaucoma. *J Ophthalmic Vis Res.* 2015;10(1):60–67.

Primary Congenital Glaucoma

Primary congenital glaucoma (PCG) accounts for the majority of primary pediatric glaucomas. Most cases are bilateral (70%) and are diagnosed within the first year of life (>75%). PCG occurs more frequently in males (65%) than females. The incidence varies with ethnicity, ranging from 1 in 1250 live births in Slovak Roms to 1 in 18,500 live births in Great Britain. Consanguinity greatly increases the risk. Without a family history of PCG, an affected parent has a 2% chance of having a child with PCG.

Newborn PCG accounts for approximately 25% of PCG cases and confers a worse prognosis than infantile PCG. More than 50% of patients with newborn PCG progress to legal blindness. The prognosis is also worse if the glaucoma is diagnosed after 1 year of age and if the corneal diameters are larger than 14 mm at diagnosis. The prognosis is best for patients whose glaucoma is diagnosed between the ages of 3 and 12 months, as most of these children respond to angle surgery.

In PCG, the pathophysiologic defect is increased resistance to outflow through the trabecular meshwork. Ophthalmologist Otto Barkan hypothesized that this resistance was caused by a membrane covering the anterior chamber angle. Although this membrane has not been identified, individuals with PCG have a developmental anomaly of the neural crest–derived tissue of the anterior chamber angle, with dysgenesis and compression of the trabecular meshwork and an anterior insertion of the iris root (Fig 6-1).

PCG in infancy presents with the classic triad of epiphora, photophobia, and blepharospasm. Until 3 years of age, elevated IOP causes the cornea to stretch, leading to increased corneal diameter and enlargement of the globe (buphthalmos). The corneal stretching produces *Haab striae,* or breaks in the Descemet membrane, and may lead to corneal edema and corneal opacification (Fig 6-2; also see Figs 22-2 and 22-3 in BCSC Section 6, *Pediatric Ophthalmology and Strabismus*). As the cornea swells, the child may become irritable and photophobic. After age 3 years, the cornea ceases to enlarge further. Scleral stretching also ceases around age 3–4 years. However, persistently elevated IOP may result in continued optic nerve damage.

The extensive differential diagnosis of PCG is presented in Table 6-3. PCG should be considered in the differential diagnosis of any child who presents with epiphora. PCG is a relatively rare disease and may go undetected or be misdiagnosed by primary care doctors

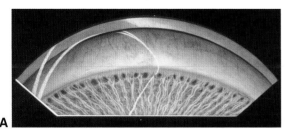 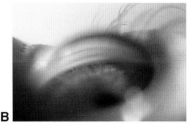

A   B

Figure 6-1   **A,** Illustration of a gonioscopic view of the anterior chamber angle in primary congenital glaucoma reveals a deep angle with no angle recess; the iris appears as a scalloped line with less density of the iris fibers (rarefaction). **B,** Goniophotograph of the angle showing a similar view. Iris blood vessels are more prominently visible in primary congenital glaucoma. *(Part A courtesy of Lee Allen and Wallace L. M. Alward, MD; part B courtesy of Robert Honkanen. MD.)*

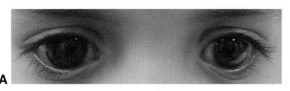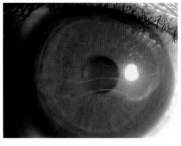

A **B**

Figure 6-2 Primary congenital glaucoma. **A,** Child with bilateral buphthalmos from uncontrolled elevated intraocular pressure prior to surgery. **B,** Photograph of Haab striae, or breaks in the Descemet membrane, which are visible after corneal edema clears. The striae are both horizontal and circumferential. *(Courtesy of Deepak Edward, MD.)*

Table 6-3 Differential Diagnosis for Symptoms and Signs of Primary Congenital Glaucoma

Conditions associated with epiphora
Nasolacrimal duct obstruction
Corneal epithelial defect or abrasion
Conjunctivitis
Keratitis
Ocular inflammation (uveitis, trauma)

Conditions associated with corneal enlargement or apparent enlargement
X-linked megalocornea
Exophthalmos
Shallow orbits (eg, craniofacial dysostoses)
Axial myopia

Conditions associated with corneal clouding
Birth trauma with breaks in Descemet membrane
Keratitis: maternal rubella, herpes, phlyctenules
Corneal dystrophies: congenital hereditary endothelial dystrophies, posterior polymorphous
    corneal dystrophy
Corneal malformations: dermoid tumors, sclerocornea, choristomas, Peters anomaly
Keratomalacia
Metabolic disorders with associated corneal abnormalities: mucopolysaccharidoses,
    sphingolipidoses, cystinoses
Skin disorders affecting the cornea: congenital ichthyosis, congenital dyskeratosis

Conditions associated with optic nerve abnormalities
Optic nerve pit
Optic nerve coloboma
Optic nerve hypoplasia
Optic nerve malformation
Optic nerve atrophy
Physiologic cupping, particularly in a large optic nerve

---

and general ophthalmologists. Mild cases may be misdiagnosed as nasolacrimal duct obstruction, resulting in a delayed PCG diagnosis and irreversible damage. Physicians must be vigilant in their examination and urgently refer infants presenting with the classic triad of epiphora, photophobia, and blepharospasm to a specialist. Left untreated, almost all cases of PCG will progress to blindness.

Treatment of PCG typically requires surgical intervention (see the Surgical Management section later in this chapter). Medical therapy has limited long-term value but may be used to temporize or reduce corneal edema to improve visualization during surgery.

Walton DS, Katsavounidou G. Newborn primary congenital glaucoma: 2005 update. *J Pediatr Ophthalmol Strabismus.* 2005;42(6):333–341.

Juvenile Open-Angle Glaucoma

Juvenile open-angle glaucoma (JOAG) is a form of primary open-angle glaucoma that presents between the ages of 4 and 35 years with elevated IOP and usually normal-appearing angles. Because most cases of JOAG are inherited as an autosomal dominant trait, many families may be aware of their risk of developing this condition, leading to earlier screening and detection. Although the IOP is elevated, it does not usually cause corneal enlargement or Haab striae due to the later age of onset; however, progressive myopia may result and continue until 10 years of age. Medical therapy is usually unsuccessful, and most patients require trabeculectomy or implantation of glaucoma tube shunts. Angle procedures may be helpful in select cases.

Developmental Glaucomas With Associated Ocular or Systemic Anomalies

The pediatric glaucomas may be associated with various ocular and systemic abnormalities, as summarized in Tables 6-1 and 6-2. The following sections discuss a few of the more common conditions.

Axenfeld-Rieger Syndrome

Axenfeld-Rieger (A-R) syndrome is a spectrum of disorders characterized by anomalous development of the neural crest–derived anterior segment structures, including the anterior chamber angle, the iris, and the trabecular meshwork. Most cases of A-R syndrome are of autosomal dominant inheritance, but sporadic cases can occur. The disorder is bilateral, with no sex predilection. Approximately 50% of cases are associated with glaucoma, typically occurring in middle or late childhood.

Although this syndrome was initially separated into Axenfeld anomaly (posterior embryotoxon with multiple adherent peripheral iris strands), Rieger anomaly (Axenfeld anomaly plus iris hypoplasia and corectopia), and Rieger syndrome (Rieger anomaly plus developmental defects of the teeth or facial bones, including maxillary hypoplasia, redundant periumbilical skin, pituitary abnormalities, or hypospadias), these disorders are now considered variations of the same clinical entity and are combined under the name *Axenfeld-Rieger syndrome.*

Classic clinical manifestations include posterior embryotoxon of the cornea (a prominent and anteriorly displaced Schwalbe line) and iris adhesions to the Schwalbe line that range from threadlike to broad bands. The iris may range from normal to markedly atrophic with corectopia, hole formation, and ectropion uveae. A-R syndrome can be distinguished from other conditions that involve abnormalities of the iris, cornea, and anterior chamber, as outlined in Table 6-4.

Peters Anomaly

Peters anomaly is a developmental condition presenting with an annular corneal opacity (leukoma) in the central visual axis, often accompanied by iris strands originating at the iris collarette and adhering to the corneal opacity. The leukoma corresponds to a defect in the corneal endothelium and underlying Descemet membrane and posterior stroma. The lens may be in its normal position, with or without a cataract, or the lens may be adherent to the posterior layers of the cornea. Patients with corneolenticular adhesions have a higher likelihood of other ocular abnormalities, such as microcornea and angle anomalies, and of systemic abnormalities, including those of the heart, genitourinary tract, musculoskeletal system, ear, palate, and spine.

Peters anomaly is usually sporadic, although autosomal dominant and autosomal recessive forms have been reported. Most cases are bilateral, and angle abnormalities leading to glaucoma occur in approximately 50% of affected patients.

The glaucoma associated with Peters anomaly is difficult to treat because of the iridocorneal dysgenesis. Angle surgery is performed if possible; alternative treatments include medications, trabeculectomy, glaucoma tube shunts, and cyclodestructive procedures.

Aniridia

Aniridia is a panocular, bilateral congenital disorder characterized by iris hypoplasia. Most patients with aniridia have only a rudimentary stump of iris; however, the iris appearance may vary greatly, with some patients having nearly complete but thin irides. Aniridia is

Table 6-4 Differential Diagnosis for Axenfeld-Rieger Syndrome

Condition	Differentiating Features
Iridocorneal endothelial syndrome	Unilateral Middle-age onset Corneal endothelial abnormalities Progressive changes
Isolated posterior embryotoxon	Lack of glaucoma-associated or iris changes
Aniridia	Iris hypoplasia Associated corneal and macular changes
Iridoschisis	Splitting of iris layers with atrophy of anterior layer
Peters anomaly	Corneal leukoma
Ectopia lentis et pupillae	Lens subluxation, pupillary displacement, axial myopia, retinal detachment, enlarged corneal diameters, cataract, prominent iris processes in the anterior chamber angle
Oculodentodigital dysplasia	Microphthalmia, microcornea, iris abnormalities, cataracts, glaucoma

associated with other ocular anomalies, including small corneas, anterior polar cataracts that may present at birth or develop later in life, and optic nerve and foveal hypoplasia resulting in pendular nystagmus and reduced vision.

In aniridia, glaucoma typically develops after the rudimentary iris stump rotates anteriorly to progressively cover the trabecular meshwork, resulting in synechial angle closure. This angle closure is a gradual process, and glaucoma may not occur until the second decade of life or later. Occasionally, however, aniridia is associated with congenital glaucoma; primary maldevelopment of the drainage angle may result in elevated IOP at a younger age.

Patients with aniridia may have limbal stem cell abnormalities that eventually result in a corneal pannus, which begins in the peripheral cornea and slowly extends centrally. There may be a role for limbal stem cell transplants in these patients.

Most cases of aniridia are familial and are transmitted with an autosomal dominant inheritance pattern; however, about one-third of cases are isolated sporadic mutations resulting from *PAX6* defects. Approximately 20% of sporadic cases are associated with a large chromosomal deletion that includes the adjacent Wilms tumor 1 gene *(WT1)*, a tumor suppressor gene, which results in an increased risk of Wilms tumor. Relatively few cases of Wilms tumor are seen in the familial form.

Two less-common forms of aniridia are associated with systemic abnormalities. *WAGR (Wilms tumor, aniridia, genitourinary anomalies, and mental retardation) syndrome* is an autosomal dominant form seen in 13% of patients with aniridia. *Gillespie syndrome* is an autosomal recessive form of aniridia associated with cerebellar ataxia and intellectual disability that occurs in 2% of those with aniridia.

Prophylactic goniosurgery may be beneficial for infants with a strong family history of aniridic glaucoma or for young children with progressive narrowing of an angle that is still open. Once the angle is closed, trabeculectomy, glaucoma tube shunts, and cyclodestruction may be required for IOP control. Thus, it is important to closely monitor the angle anatomy with serial gonioscopy.

Sturge-Weber Syndrome

Sturge-Weber syndrome (SWS; also known as *encephalotrigeminal angiomatosis*) is a phakomatosis with ipsilateral facial cutaneous hemangioma (nevus flammeus or port-wine stain), ipsilateral choroidal cavernous hemangioma (tomato ketchup fundus), and ipsilateral leptomeningeal angioma associated with cerebral calcifications, seizures, focal neurologic deficits, and a variable degree of cognitive impairment. The condition is usually unilateral but can present bilaterally in rare instances. There is no race or sex predilection, and no inheritance pattern has been established. Glaucoma occurs in 30%–70% of children with SWS and is more common when the nevus flammeus involves the eyelids. When seen in infants with this syndrome, the glaucoma is thought to be due to congenital anterior chamber anomalies (similar to PCG). Glaucoma that develops after the first decade of life may be caused by elevated episcleral venous pressure. Trabeculectomy should be performed with caution because of an increased risk of choroidal effusion and choroidal hemorrhage in these patients.

Neurofibromatosis

Neurofibromatosis (NF), the most common phakomatosis, has 2 recognizable forms. Neurofibromatosis 1 (NF1), also known as *von Recklinghausen disease* or *peripheral neurofibromatosis,* is the most common type, with a prevalence of 1 in 3000–5000 persons. NF1 is localized to band 11 of the long arm of chromosome 17 and is inherited in an autosomal dominant fashion in approximately 50% of cases; the other 50% of cases are sporadic. Ectropion uveae is a common ocular finding whose presence in a neonate should prompt a workup for NF1. Other ocular findings associated with NF1 include Lisch nodules, optic nerve gliomas, eyelid neurofibromas, and glaucoma. Systemic findings include cutaneous café-au-lait spots, cutaneous neurofibromas, and axillary or inguinal freckling.

Neurofibromatosis 2, or *central neurofibromatosis,* is defined by the presence of bilateral acoustic neuromas and is not associated with glaucoma.

Secondary Glaucomas

Many of the causes of secondary glaucoma in infants and children are similar to those in adults (see Table 6-2), including trauma, inflammation, steroid use, and topiramate-induced angle closure. Lens-associated disorders causing angle-closure glaucoma may occur in patients with Marfan syndrome, homocystinuria, Weill-Marchesani syndrome, and microspherophakia. Posterior segment disorders such as persistent fetal vasculature, retinopathy of prematurity, and familial exudative vitreoretinopathy, as well as tumors of the retina, iris, or ciliary body, can also result in glaucoma. Retinoblastoma, juvenile xanthogranuloma, and medulloepithelioma are some of the intraocular tumors known to lead to secondary glaucoma in infants and children. Rubella and congenital cataract are important conditions that are also associated with secondary pediatric glaucoma.

Aphakic Glaucoma

Glaucoma develops in 15%–50% or more of children who have undergone surgery for congenital cataract. Risk factors for aphakic glaucoma include cataract surgery in the first year of life, postoperative complications, and small corneal diameter. Although most aphakic glaucoma develops in patients within 3 years of cataract surgery, these patients are always at risk for glaucoma and thus require lifelong follow-up. The underlying mechanism is unclear, but likely etiologies include congenital anomalies, surgically induced inflammation, and altered intraocular anatomy postoperatively. Removing all residual cortex during cataract surgery may reduce the occurrence of pediatric aphakic glaucoma.

Aponte EP, Diehl N, Mohney BG. Incidence and clinical characteristics of childhood glaucoma: a population-based study. *Arch Ophthalmol.* 2010;128(4):478–482.

Chen TC, Bhatia LS, Halpern EF, Walton DS. Risk factors for the development of aphakic glaucoma after congenital cataract surgery. *J Pediatr Ophthalmol Strabismus.* 2006;43(5): 274–280.

Papadopoulos M, Cable N, Rahi J, Khaw PT; BIG Eye Study Investigators. The British Infantile and Childhood Glaucoma (BIG) Eye Study. *Invest Ophthalmol Vis Sci.* 2007; 48(9):4100–4106.

Yanovitch TL, Freedman SF. Pediatric glaucoma. *Focal Points: Clinical Modules for Ophthalmologists.* San Francisco: American Academy of Ophthalmology; 2012, module 3.

Evaluating the Pediatric Glaucoma Patient

A pediatric glaucoma patient should be evaluated differently than an adult with glaucoma. Ophthalmologists should proceed with an orderly system of examination and the appropriate equipment for evaluating infants and young children in both the office and the operating room (Table 6-5). For examinations under anesthesia (EUAs), efficiency in measuring and recording data in the operating room can minimize the time that the patient is under anesthesia.

History

When evaluating an infant, the ophthalmologist should ask the caregiver whether the baby is fussy or irritable, whether the child is not feeding well or is losing weight, and whether the baby cries when taken outside into sunshine. The caregiver's observations regarding any corneal clouding should be sought, specifically as to whether the clouding is intermittent or constant.

For evaluation of school-aged children, the ophthalmologist should inquire about the results of school vision screenings, changes in academic performance, and complaints about trouble seeing in the classroom. A complete record of the patient's history should include the names of previous physicians who have been consulted; all prior ocular and systemic medical and surgical treatments; any family history of congenital glaucoma and other ocular and systemic disorders; medication use (with particular attention to all forms of steroids); and allergies.

Table 6-5 Supplies for Examining Children Under Anesthesia

Examination form/checklist
Topical medications
  Anesthetics
  Mydriatics (use only if not proceeding with angle surgery)
  Coupling or balanced salt solution for gonioscopy
  Glycerol
  Pilocarpine and apraclonidine if proceeding with angle surgery
Tonometer: Tono-Pen, Perkins, or pneumatonometer
Calipers
Koeppe or other angle lens
Direct ophthalmoscope
Portable slit lamp
A-scan ultrasonography system
B-scan ultrasonography system
Retinoscope and lenses for refraction
Indirect ophthalmoscope and lens
Pachymeter
Portable fundus camera

Visual Acuity

Testing of visual acuity in infants and young children is discussed in BCSC Section 6, *Pediatric Ophthalmology and Strabismus.* Refraction should be performed to identify any myopia from axial enlargement, and/or astigmatism from corneal irregularity. Decreased vision may be due to significant glaucomatous optic nerve damage, amblyopia, corneal scarring, or other associated ocular disorders (eg, retinal detachment, macular edema, cataract, lens dislocation).

External Examination

The ophthalmologist should look for buphthalmos (see Fig 6-2) and other signs and symptoms of PCG, including epiphora and blepharospasm, as well as features that may be associated with primary and secondary glaucomas other than PCG. These features include chromosomal abnormalities, phakomatoses, connective tissue disorders, and A-R syndrome.

Anterior Segment Examination

As discussed previously, corneal enlargement and opacification are important signs associated with glaucoma in patients younger than 3 years. Corneal diameter should be measured with calipers or a ruler. The normal corneal diameter is approximately 9.5–10.5 mm in full-term newborns, increasing to 11–12 mm by 1 year of age. In contrast, eyes with congenital glaucoma may have a corneal diameter greater than 12 mm in the first year of life. Corneal edema may be due to elevated IOP or Haab striae and may range from mild haze to dense opacification of the corneal stroma (see Fig 6-2). Retroillumination after pupillary dilation may help make Haab striae visible. Evaluation for other anterior segment anomalies, such as aniridia, iridocorneal adhesions, and corectopia, may provide insight into the underlying diagnosis.

Tonometry

Accurate tonometry is vital in the assessment of the pediatric glaucomas. IOP may be falsely elevated in an uncooperative or struggling child. Often, the clinician can successfully measure the IOP of an infant younger than 6 months without general anesthesia or sedation by performing the measurement while the infant is feeding or immediately thereafter. For this group of patients, the Tono-Pen (Reichert Ophthalmic Instruments, Depew, NY) or pneumatonometer works best for in-office tonometry. The Perkins tonometer can also be helpful for children who are too young to cooperate for Goldmann tonometry at the slit lamp. The rebound tonometer, a newer instrument that does not require topical anesthesia, is playing a greater role in the office because it can decrease the need for EUAs when obtaining IOP. It also can be used for measuring IOP in the pediatric patient's home. However, despite these advantages, initial reports indicate that measurements in patients with congenital glaucoma were higher with the rebound tonometer than with the Perkins tonometer.

General anesthesia is usually required for accurate IOP assessment of older infants (≥6 months) and young children. However, most general anesthetic agents and sedatives can profoundly lower IOP. Exceptions include chloral hydrate, which does not affect IOP, and ketamine, which may increase IOP. In addition, the preparation for general anesthesia may cause infants to become dehydrated, which can reduce IOP. Increased IOP during general anesthesia may result from endotracheal intubation, upward drift of the eyes, or possible induced laryngospasm. It is best to coordinate with the anesthesiologist before the child is brought to the operating room and arrange to take the IOP measurement immediately after induction of general anesthesia (preferably before intubation), which should minimize the effects of anesthesia on IOP.

Normal IOP in newborns is in the low teens; by middle childhood, IOP increases to adult levels of 10–20 mm Hg. Glaucoma should be suspected if IOPs are elevated or asymmetric in a cooperative or anesthetized child.

Martinez-de-la-Casa JM, Garcia-Feijoo J, Saenz-Frances F, et al. Comparison of rebound tonometer and Goldmann handheld applanation tonometer in congenital glaucoma. *J Glaucoma.* 2009;18(1):49–52.

Pachymetry

The role of pachymetry in the diagnosis and management of pediatric glaucoma is unclear. The average central corneal thickness (CCT) is 540–560 μm in children without glaucoma. CCT is lower than average in eyes with congenital glaucoma and in children with Down syndrome; CCT is higher than average in eyes with aphakic glaucoma and aniridia. It is also slightly higher in premature infants. The effect of CCT on the accuracy of IOP measurements in these groups is unclear, and nomograms cannot accurately be used to "correct" IOP measurements for differences in CCT measurements.

Bradfield YS, Melia BM, Repka MX, et al; Pediatric Eye Disease Investigator Group. Central corneal thickness in children. *Arch Ophthalmol.* 2011;129(9):1132–1138.
Tai TY, Mills MD, Beck AD, et al. Central corneal thickness and corneal diameter in patients with childhood glaucoma. *J Glaucoma.* 2006;15(6):524–528.

Gonioscopy

Gonioscopy provides important information about the mechanism of the pediatric glaucoma as well as evidence of a patient's prior surgeries. An EUA is usually required for gonioscopic examination of younger children. A Koeppe lens allows direct visualization of the angle structures. In older children, indirect gonioscopy can be performed with a 4-mirror goniolens at the slit lamp.

The normal anterior chamber angle of an infant differs from the normal adult angle in several ways, including a less pigmented trabecular meshwork, a less prominent Schwalbe line, and a less distinct junction between the scleral spur and ciliary body band. In PCG, the anterior chamber is deep, with a high anterior iris insertion. The angle recess is absent, and the iris root appears as a scalloped line of glistening tissue. Although this tissue is not a true membrane, it has been referred to as the *Barkan membrane* and likely represents thickened and compacted trabecular meshwork (see Fig 6-1).

In JOAG, the angle usually appears normal. In aniridia, gonioscopy reveals a rudimentary iris root with progressive narrowing of the angle that eventually results in synechial closure.

Optic Nerve and Fundus Evaluation

Visualization and documentation of the optic nerve are crucial to the evaluation and management of pediatric glaucomas. Evaluation of the optic nerve is often performed with direct ophthalmoscopy, which can be done in the office or operating room. Alternatively, indirect ophthalmoscopy can be used. In patients with small pupils, viewing can be enhanced through a Koeppe lens without a dimple. In older children, slit-lamp biomicroscopy can be performed. Photographs provide the best documentation and help the ophthalmologist evaluate changes over time.

A typical newborn without glaucoma has a small physiologic cup (cup–disc ratio [CDR] less than 0.3) with a pink rim. In PCG, the optic canal is stretched and the lamina cribrosa is bowed backward, causing generalized enlargement of the cup. Enlarged or increasing CDR or CDR asymmetry greater than 0.2 between the 2 eyes is suggestive of glaucomatous cupping. Cupping may be reversible if the IOP is lowered; however, lowering IOP cannot reverse any existing atrophy of the optic nerve axons.

A-Scan Ultrasonography

Serial measurements of axial length using A-scan ultrasonography can document progressive globe enlargement in patients with PCG. Axial length may stabilize or decrease with control of IOP and thus serves as a critical marker for successful control of IOP.

Law SK, Bui D, Caprioli J. Serial axial length measurement in congenital glaucoma. *Am J Ophthalmol.* 2001;132(6):926.

Other Testing

B-scan ultrasonography should be performed if media opacities, particularly corneal edema, preclude fundus evaluation. Scanning laser ophthalmoscopy and optical coherence tomography can provide useful longitudinal data in older children with clear media; however, no normative databases are available for children.

Treatment Overview

Surgical Management

Surgery is the preferred, definitive treatment of most cases of PCG; medications have limited long-term value. In other forms of pediatric glaucoma, medication can better control IOP, but a high percentage of these cases also eventually require surgery. Goniotomy and ab externo trabeculotomy are the procedures of choice for the treatment of PCG. Either procedure is appropriate if the cornea is clear. If the cornea is cloudy, goniotomy is difficult because of poor visualization of the target structures; trabeculotomy is thus more easily performed. In patients with clear corneas, angle surgery with either of these procedures yields a 70%–80% success rate in children with PCG diagnosed between 3 and 12 months of age. Angle surgery may also be used to treat other forms of pediatric glaucoma, including glaucoma associated with aniridia, A-R syndrome, or Sturge-Weber syndrome.

Trabeculectomy and glaucoma tube shunt implantation should be reserved for congenital glaucoma cases in which goniotomy or trabeculotomy has failed or for treatment of other forms of pediatric glaucoma. Cyclodestruction is necessary in some intractable cases, but because of the risk of phthisis bulbi, it should be avoided if possible.

Glaucoma surgery in children poses unique difficulties. For example, in PCG, the anatomical landmarks are distorted in the buphthalmic eye, and the thin sclera presents additional difficulties during trabeculotomy and trabeculectomy. The surgeon performing glaucoma surgery in pediatric patients should be experienced in handling these challenges and able to provide the necessary environment for evaluating these patients postoperatively. Additional surgery is often required, so the surgeon should also develop a long-term plan in order to keep surgical options available for the future and to minimize the risk of visual compromise.

The decision to proceed with angle surgery is often made during an EUA; ideally, if glaucoma is diagnosed, angle surgery should be performed during the same anesthesia session in order to minimize the number of general anesthesia sessions for the child. If angle surgery is anticipated, it is best not to dilate the eye during the EUA in order to protect the lens during the surgical procedure.

In a goniotomy, the angle is visualized with a surgical gonioscopic contact lens, a needle knife is passed across the anterior chamber, and a superficial incision is made in the uveal trabecular meshwork (Fig 6-3). A clear cornea is required in order to visualize the angle.

In a trabeculotomy, the Schlemm canal is cannulated from an external approach, and the trabecular meshwork is opened by breaking through the Schlemm canal into the anterior chamber. The procedure begins with creation of a conjunctival flap, beneath which a partial-thickness scleral flap is created, similar to a trabeculectomy. Beneath that

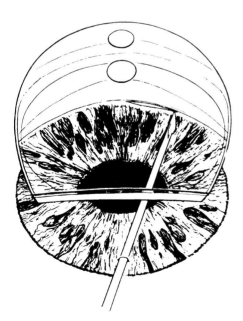

Figure 6-3 Illustration of a goniotomy incision as seen through a surgical contact lens.

partial-thickness scleral flap, the surgeon identifies the Schlemm canal, either by creating a radial incision into the sclera or by dissecting a deep scleral flap and noting the canal at the edges of this flap. Alternatively, the surgeon can identify the canal edges after unroofing the Schlemm canal by creating a single deep scleral flap. The surgeon inserts a fine wirelike instrument (trabeculotome) into the Schlemm canal and then rotates it into the anterior chamber, tearing the trabecular meshwork (Fig 6-4). Alternatively, a 6-0 nonabsorbable polypropylene suture can be fed through the Schlemm canal for its entire 360° circumference and pulled tautly into the anterior chamber. When using either the trabeculotome or the suture, the surgeon must take care to avoid creating a false passage or entering the subretinal or suprachoroidal spaces.

Another option in trabeculotomy is the use of a fiber-optic microcatheter to cannulate the Schlemm canal until the cannula passes through 360°. The ends of the catheter can then be grasped and pulled in opposite directions to perform a 360° trabeculotomy. An advantage of using this catheter is that the surgeon knows where the leading catheter tip is at all times because of the red light that illuminates it (see Chapter 8, Video 8-6).

Many surgeons inject viscoelastic into the anterior chamber at the start of goniotomy and trabeculotomy in order to prevent collapse of the chamber and to tamponade bleeding

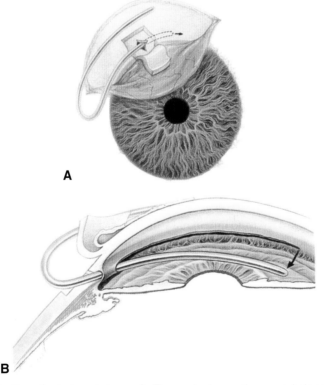

A

B

Figure 6-4 Illustration of a trabeculotomy. **A,** The probe is gently passed along the Schlemm canal, with little resistance for 6–10 mm. **B,** By rotating the probe internally *(arrow)*, the surgeon ruptures the trabecular meshwork and the probe appears in the anterior chamber with minimal bleeding. *(Reproduced and modified with permission from Kolker AE, Hetherington J, eds.* Becker-Shaffer's Diagnosis and Therapy of the Glaucomas. *5th ed. St Louis: Mosby; 1983.)*

intraoperatively. Thorough removal of the viscoelastic at the end of the procedure is nec-essary to prevent a postoperative spike in IOP.

The success rates of these 2 angle surgeries are similar, but each procedure has its ad-vantages and disadvantages. When the cornea is clear, goniotomy has the following advan-tages over trabeculotomy: there is no postoperative conjunctival scarring (scarring could limit future filtering surgery); the procedure is much faster; and there is less trauma to the anterior segment tissues. Trabeculotomy offers the following advantages: the approach to trabeculotomy is more familiar to surgeons experienced in adult glaucoma procedures; it can be performed in an opacified cornea; and it can be converted to a trabeculectomy if the Schlemm canal cannot be cannulated.

Complications associated with these procedures include hyphema, infection, lens damage, and uveitis. The Descemet membrane may be stripped during a trabeculotomy. General anesthesia may cause serious complications in children; to minimize these risks bilateral procedures are performed in some children.

Angle surgery has a success rate of 70%–80% in infants presenting with PCG between 3 and 12 months of age; this success rate includes repeated angle procedures, which is common in this disease. Trabeculectomy or implantation of a glaucoma tube shunt should be considered when 2 or more angle surgeries are not successful in lowering the IOP or when adjunctive medical therapy is inadequate. Surgeons should also consider these op-tions for children who have forms of glaucoma other than PCG, although angle surgery is often successful in aphakic glaucoma and in new onset of glaucoma associated with aniridia.

If angle surgery is not successful, the surgeon must take several factors into account when deciding between trabeculectomy and implantation of a glaucoma tube shunt as the next procedure. Trabeculectomy has a low success rate in children younger than 2 years and in aphakic eyes. Bleb scarring and failure are very prevalent without the use of antifibrotics, but there are serious risks of bleb leaks and bleb infections with the use of these agents. To avoid the risk of blebitis and endophthalmitis, mitomycin C (MMC)–augmented trabeculectomy should be performed with caution in pediatric pa-tients who are too young to understand good hygiene, which is necessary to minimize the chances of infection.

Glaucoma tube shunts are useful for lowering IOP and lack the risk of bleb-related infections. Success rates vary with different tube shunts, diagnoses, and patient ages. Complications include anterior migration of the tube shunt with resultant corneal dam-age, tube blockage, tube erosion with resultant endophthalmitis, cataract, motility distur-bances, bleb encapsulation with elevated IOP, and pupil distortion. The IOPs are usually higher after implantation of these devices than after successful trabeculectomy, and most of the children who have undergone implantation will need to continue using topical glau-coma medications. The various styles and sizes of glaucoma tube shunts can help indi-vidualize the surgery to the patient's situation.

Cyclodestruction is reserved for cases refractory to other surgical and medical treatments. Cyclodestructive procedures lower IOP by causing areas of the ciliary body to atrophy, resulting in less aqueous production. Cyclodestructive techniques include cyclocryotherapy, transscleral cyclophotocoagulation (CPC) with the Nd:YAG or diode laser, and endoscopic cyclophotocoagulation (ECP). When these techniques are used in pediatric patients, general anesthesia is required. The rate of complications is lower with cyclodestructive laser procedures than with cryotherapy. One disadvantage of cyclodestructive procedures is the difficulty in titrating the results. Another disadvantage is the serious potential complications—which include hypotony, uveitis, retinal detachment, phthisis bulbi, and blindness. The most common cyclodestructive modalities currently used are transscleral CPC with the diode laser and ECP. Transscleral CPC is a noninvasive procedure, whereas ECP is an intraocular procedure in which the laser energy is applied under direct visualization, causing less damage to adjacent tissues. ECP is particularly useful in eyes with distorted anterior segment anatomy and in eyes with prior unsuccessful CPC or cryotherapy. Transscleral CPC and ECP can be very useful for providing additional IOP lowering after glaucoma tube shunt surgery.

Barkan O. Goniotomy for the relief of congenital glaucoma. *Br J Ophthalmol.* 1948;32(9): 701–728.

Beck AD, Lynch MG. 360 degrees trabeculotomy for primary congenital glaucoma. *Arch Ophthalmol.* 1995;113(9):1200–1202.

Bothun ED, Guo Y, Christiansen SP, et al. Outcome of angle surgery in children with aphakic glaucoma. *J AAPOS.* 2010;14(3):235–239.

Girkin CA, Rhodes L, McGwin G, Marchase N, Cogen MS. Goniotomy versus circumferential trabeculotomy with an illuminated micro catheter in congenital glaucoma. *J AAPOS.* 2012; 16(5):424–427.

Neely DE, Plager DA. Endocyclophotocoagulation for management of difficult pediatric glaucomas. *J AAPOS.* 2001;5(4):221–229.

O'Malley Schotthoefer E, Yanovitch TL, Freedman SF. Aqueous drainage device surgery in refractory pediatric glaucomas: I. Long-term outcomes. *J AAPOS.* 2008;12(1):33–39.

O'Malley Schotthoefer E, Yanovitch TL, Freedman SF. Aqueous drainage device surgery in refractory pediatric glaucoma: II. Ocular motility consequences. *J AAPOS.* 2008;12(1): 40–45.

Medical Management

Although surgical management is the foundation of PCG care, medications are frequently required in the treatment of PCG and other pediatric glaucomas. Medications can be used to lower IOP before surgery in order to reduce corneal edema and improve visualization during surgery. They may also be used after surgical procedures in order to provide additional IOP lowering. Medical therapy may also be useful in treating JOAG, inflammatory glaucoma, and aphakic glaucoma and other secondary glaucomas. The safety and efficacy of most FDA-approved glaucoma medications have not been studied in controlled clinical trials specifically in children, although most clinicians are guided by extensive clinical experience. When the patient is a preadolescent or adolescent female, clinicians must inquire about pregnancy before initiating any treatment that might affect a fetus. A full discussion of glaucoma medications can be found in Chapter 7.

β-Adrenergic antagonists

β-Adrenergic antagonists, or β-blockers, decrease aqueous production in the ciliary body and thus can be useful for controlling IOP in children. Topical β-blockers, topical carbonic anhydrase inhibitors, and prostaglandin analogues are reasonable first-line agents in children. These agents must be used with caution, however. The systemic absorption of these agents is considerable—even with topical application—and can cause bronchospasm, bradycardia, and hypotension in susceptible children. β-Blockers should thus be avoided in children with asthma or significant cardiac disease. To decrease the risk of bronchospasm, the clinician may consider administering the cardioselective β-blocker betaxolol. The risk of adverse effects can also be diminished with occlusion of the nasolacrimal drainage system for 3 minutes after administration and use of a lower dose (eg, timolol 0.25% or levobunolol 0.25% as opposed to 0.5%), particularly for young children. The clinician should teach parents how to occlude the nasolacrimal drainage system for administration at home. Patients with lighter irides may respond as well to timolol 0.25% or levobunolol 0.25% as they do to 0.5% of the same medications.

Carbonic anhydrase inhibitors

Like β-adrenergic antagonists, carbonic anhydrase inhibitors (CAIs) decrease IOP by reducing aqueous production. Topical use of dorzolamide or brinzolamide has a minimal risk of systemic adverse effects and is also an excellent first-line therapy. Systemic CAIs (acetazolamide and methazolamide) provide slightly more IOP lowering than the topical preparations but have numerous systemic adverse effects. The pediatric dosage of acetazolamide is 10–20 mg/kg/day. CAIs should not be used in patients with known serious sulfa allergies. Adverse effects of CAIs include anorexia, diarrhea, weight loss, tingling of the perioral areas and fingers, hypokalemia, metabolic acidosis, which can affect bone growth, and risk of sickle cell crisis in sickle cell anemia; children using diuretics are particularly at risk for these adverse effects. Because of the risk of these effects and of rare but life-threatening reactions such as Stevens-Johnson syndrome and aplastic anemia, systemic CAIs are reserved for patients at great risk of vision loss due to highly elevated IOP.

α-Adrenergic agonists

α-Adrenergic agonists lower IOP by diminishing aqueous production and increasing uveoscleral outflow. The α_2-adrenergic agonist brimonidine, which crosses the blood–brain barrier, may have significant effects on the central nervous system, including apnea, hypotension, bradycardia, hypotonia, hypothermia, and somnolence. Infants and young children are particularly susceptible to brimonidine's adverse effects; thus α_2-adrenergic agonists are contraindicated in children younger than 3 years. There is some debate about the age at which children can safely use brimonidine. In general, it should be used with caution in children between the ages of 3 and 10 years old. The lowest dose possible should be used and punctal occlusion employed to minimize systemic absorption.

The α-adrenergic agonist apraclonidine is better tolerated systemically in children, but the risk of follicular conjunctivitis increases with long-term use. Apraclonidine also acts as a vasoconstrictor and can be used to minimize bleeding during intraocular surgery.

Prostaglandin analogues

Prostaglandin analogues lower IOP by increasing uveoscleral outflow. They have minimal systemic side effects in children and have been shown to effectively lower IOP in JOAG.

However, they can exacerbate uveitis in postoperative glaucoma patients, so they should be avoided in patients with uncontrolled uveitis. Their once-daily dosing can help minimize the stress involved in administering eyedrops to children. Adverse effects include conjunctival hyperemia, hypertrichosis and trichiasis, periocular pigmentation (reversible), and permanent darkening of irides, except in blue-eyed patients.

Cholinergic agonists

Cholinergic agonists (miotics) lower IOP by increasing aqueous outflow through the trabecular meshwork. Because newer medications are available, these agents are rarely used on a long-term basis. However, they have a role intraoperatively by inducing miosis, which facilitates angle surgery.

Chang L, Ong EL, Bunce C, Brookes J, Papadopoulos M, Khaw PT. A review of the medical treatment of pediatric glaucomas at Moorsfield eye hospital. *J Glaucoma.* 2013;22(8): 601–607.

Coppens G, Stalmans I, Zeyen T, Casteels I. The safety and efficacy of glaucoma medications in the pediatric population. *J Pediatr Ophthalmol Strabismus.* 2009;46(1):12–18.

Maeda-Chubachi TM, Chi-Burns K, Simons D, et al. Comparison of latanoprost and timolol in pediatric glaucoma: a phase 3, 12-week, randomized, double-masked multicenter study. *Ophthalmology.* 2011;118(10):2014–2021.

Prognosis and Follow-Up

The development of effective surgical techniques has greatly improved the long-term prognosis for pediatric glaucoma patients, particularly PCG patients asymptomatic at birth who present with onset of symptoms between 3 and 12 months of age. These patients have a good prognosis, although multiple surgeries may be required. When symptoms are present at birth or when the disease is diagnosed after 12 months of age, the prognosis for surgical control of IOP is poor.

Pediatric patients whose IOP is controlled by surgery may still experience morbidities related to previous IOP elevation, including amblyopia, corneal scarring, strabismus, anisometropia, cataract, lens subluxation, susceptibility to trauma (eg, as in an eye with a thinned sclera), and recurrent glaucoma in the affected or unaffected eye. These morbidities can cause serious long-term visual compromise and thus should be addressed by clinicians promptly.

Amblyopia is a common cause of visual compromise, particularly in patients with unilateral glaucoma, corneal opacification, and/or anisometropia. The clinician should treat amblyopia aggressively, addressing conditions contributing to its development, such as refractive error, strabismus, cataract, and corneal clouding. Elevated IOP can lead to buphthalmos in patients with PCG and to progressive myopia and anisometropia in patients with JOAG. Haab striae and corneal scarring may cause astigmatism. Refractive errors should be corrected with spectacles, and use of protective eyewear should be encouraged.

Strabismus may result from glaucoma tube shunts or amblyopia. When performing surgery to correct strabismus, the surgeon should try to minimize conjunctival scarring in anticipation of future glaucoma surgeries and should be cognizant of the sites of prior trabeculectomies and glaucoma tube shunt implants.

All cases of pediatric glaucoma require lifelong follow-up to monitor IOP, potential complications from prior surgeries, and secondary vision-threatening issues. Because relapses of glaucoma may occur even years later, glaucoma specialists and pediatric specialists should coordinate care. Educating parents about the need for lifelong care of the child with glaucoma and involving these children in their own care enhance the long-term management of this challenging disease.

de Silva DJ, Khaw PT, Brookes JL. Long-term outcome of primary congenital glaucoma. *J AAPOS*. 2011;15(2):148–152.

Khitri MR, Mills MD, Ying GS, Davidson SL, Quinn GE. Visual acuity outcomes in pediatric glaucomas. *J AAPOS*. 2012;16(4):376–381.

CHAPTER 7

Medical Management of Glaucoma

The goal of currently available glaucoma therapy is to preserve visual function by lowering intraocular pressure (IOP) to a level that is likely to prevent further optic nerve damage. The treatment regimen chosen should achieve this goal with the lowest risk, fewest adverse effects, and the least amount of disruption to the patient's life, taking into account the cost of treatment. Although the goal of treatment is to prevent vision loss, current treatments are aimed at lowering IOP and, in the short term, the efficacy of treatment is gauged according to the IOP level.

The *target pressure* is an IOP range below which the clinician estimates the risk of disease progression is sufficiently low so as to minimize the patient's risk of experiencing further symptomatic vision loss in his or her lifetime. It should be individualized for the patient, based on the following: IOP level at which damage is thought to have occurred; severity of the damage; the previously observed rate of progression (if known); life expectancy of the patient; and risk factors such as a history of disc hemorrhages, high myopia, a thinner cornea, and a family history of severe vision loss in the setting of glaucoma (risk factors are discussed in more detail in Chapter 4).

The more advanced the disease on initial presentation, the lower the target pressure required for preventing further progression in the average patient. Evidence suggests that the severity of optic nerve injury may increase the likelihood of continued disease progression. Furthermore, if severe vision loss is already present, further damage is likely to have a disproportionately greater impact on visual function and quality of life. A reduction in IOP of at least 25% below baseline is a reasonable initial target for most patients with mild to moderate damage. However, there is no guarantee that reducing IOP to the target pressure will prevent disease progression. If further progression does occur, the target pressure may require downward revision.

After determining the target pressure, the clinician must decide whether to achieve this goal medically or surgically. Regardless of which option the clinician chooses, the anticipated benefits of any therapeutic regimen should justify the risks; regimens associated with substantial adverse effects should be reserved for patients with a high probability of progressive vision loss. Sometimes it may be necessary to accept an IOP level above the established target pressure because the adverse effects or risks of intensified therapy may be unacceptable. The clinician must consider both the impact of treatment and the impact of the disease on the patient's overall quality of life.

Initial treatment of ocular hypertension (defined in Chapter 4) and most glaucomas typically involves drugs. When starting patients on a medication, some clinicians use a unilateral treatment trial to assess the drug's efficacy; however, evidence suggests this may be of limited value because of the occurrence of asymmetric IOP fluctuation between fellow eyes. Ocular hypotensive agents are divided into several classes based on chemical structure and pharmacologic action. Classes in common clinical use include

- prostaglandin analogues
- adrenergic drugs, divided into β-adrenergic antagonists and adrenergic agonists
- carbonic anhydrase inhibitors (topical and systemic)
- parasympathomimetic (miotic) agents, including direct-acting cholinergic agonists and indirect-acting anticholinesterase agents
- combination medications
- hyperosmotic agents

Table 7-1 lists the various glaucoma medications (updated version at www.aao.org/bcsc _s10_table7-1). See BCSC Section 2, *Fundamentals and Principles of Ophthalmology,* for further discussion of the mechanisms of action of these drugs.

> Netland PA, ed. *Glaucoma Medical Therapy: Principles and Management.* 2nd ed. Ophthalmology Monographs 13. New York: Oxford University Press; 2007.

Prostaglandin Analogues

Mechanism of Action

Ocular hypotensive prostaglandin analogues are prodrugs that penetrate the cornea and become biologically active after being hydrolyzed by corneal esterase. They lower IOP by increasing outflow via the uveoscleral pathway and, to a variable extent, decreasing outflow resistance. The precise mechanism by which these changes occur has not been fully determined. It is thought that these drugs bind to various prostaglandin receptors, most importantly prostaglandin $F_{2\alpha}$ ($PGF_{2\alpha}$), triggering a cascade of events that leads to activation of matrix metalloproteinases. This in turn leads to remodeling of the ciliary body, trabecular meshwork, and possibly scleral extracellular matrix, such that the volume of aqueous able to flow directly through these tissues is increased. Topical therapy results in increased space between the muscle fascicles within the ciliary body, thought to be the main site of uveoscleral outflow. Latanoprostene bunod—a new, chemically modified prostaglandin analogue with a nitric oxide-donating moiety—has been found to be slightly more effective than latanoprost, presumably because nitric oxide acts on the meshwork and Schlemm canal to improve trabecular outflow facility.

Available Agents and Dosing Frequency

Currently, 4 prostaglandin analogues are in widespread clinical use: latanoprost, travoprost, bimatoprost, and tafluprost. Both latanoprost and travoprost reduce IOP by 25%–32%; bimatoprost lowers IOP by 27%–33%. Tafluprost, currently the only preservative-free

Table 7-1 Glaucoma Medications

Class/Compound	Concentration	Dosing	Mechanism of Action	IOP Reduction	Ocular	Systemic	Comments, Including Time to Peak Effect and Washout
					Adverse Effects		
Prostaglandin analogues							
Latanoprost	0.005%	Once daily	Increases uveoscleral outflow primarily. Also increases conventional outflow.	25%–32%	Increased pigmentation of iris and lashes, hypertrichosis, trichiasis, distichiasis, blurred vision, keratitis, anterior uveitis, conjunctival hyperemia, exacerbation of herpes keratitis, CME, prostaglandin-associated periorbitopathy	Flulike symptoms, joint/muscle pain, headache	±IOP-lowering effect with miotic Peak: 10–14 hours Washout: 4–6 weeks Maximum IOP-lowering effect may take up to 6 weeks to occur
Travoprost	0.004%	Once daily	Same as above	25%–32%	Same as above	Same as above	Same as above
Bimatoprost	0.03, 0.01%	Once daily	Same as above	27%–33%	Same as above	Same as above	Same as above
Tafluprost	0.0015%	Once daily	Increases uveoscleral outflow	27%–31%	Same as above	Same as above	Same as above
β-Adrenergic antagonists (β-blockers)							
Nonselective							
Timolol maleate	0.25% and 0.50% solution or gel Also 0.1% gel	Solutions: 1–2 times daily Gels: once daily	Decreases aqueous production	20%–30%	Blurring, irritation, corneal anesthesia, punctate keratitis, allergy; aggravation of myasthenia gravis	Bradycardia, heart block, bronchospasm, lowered blood pressure, decreased libido, CNS depression, mood swings, reduced exercise tolerance, masked symptoms of hypoglycemia, exacerbation of myasthenia gravis	May be less effective if patient is taking systemic β-blockers; short-term escape, long-term drift; diabetic patients may experience reduced glucose tolerance and masking of hypoglycemic signs/symptoms Peak: 2–3 hours Washout: 1 month
Timolol hemihydrate	0.5%	As above	Same as above	20%–30%	Same as above	Same as above	—
Levobunolol	0.25, 0.5%	As above	Same as above	20%–30%	Same as above	Same as above	Peak: 2–6 hours
Metipranolol	0.3%	2 times daily	Same as above	20%–30%	Same as above	Same as above	Report of iritis Peak: 2 hours
Carteolol hydrochloride	1.0%	1–2 times daily	—	—	—	Intrinsic sympathomimetic	May have less effect on nocturnal pulse, blood pressure Peak: 4 hours Washout: 1 month

(Continued)

Class/Compound	Concentration	Dosing	Mechanism of Action	IOP Reduction	Adverse Effects		Comments, Including Time to Peak Effect and Washout
					Ocular	Systemic	
Selective							
Betaxolol	0.25%	2 times daily	Same as above	15%–20%	Same as above	Lower risk of pulmonary complications	Peak: 2–3 hours Washout: 1 month
α₂-Adrenergic agonists							
Selective							
Apraclonidine hydrochloride	0.5, 1.0%	2–3 times daily	Decreases aqueous production	20%–30%	Irritation, ischemia, allergy, eyelid retraction, conjunctival blanching, follicular conjunctivitis, pruritus, dermatitis, ocular ache, photopsia, miosis	Hypotension, vasovagal attack, dry mouth and nose, fatigue	Useful in pre- or postlaser or cataract surgery Tachyphylaxis may limit long-term use. Peak: <1–2 hours Washout: 7–14 days
Brimonidine tartrate 0.2%	0.2%	2–3 times daily	Decreases aqueous production, increases uveoscleral outflow	20%–30%	Blurring, foreign-body sensation, eyelid edema, dryness, less ocular sensitivity/allergy than with apraclonidine	Headache, fatigue, hypotension, insomnia, depression, syncope, dizziness, anxiety, dry mouth	Highly selective for α₂-receptor Brimonidine should not be used in infants and young children. Peak: 2 hours Washout: 7–14 days
Brimonidine tartrate in Purite 0.1%	0.1%	2–3 times daily	Same as above	Same as above	Same as above, except less allergy than with brimonidine 0.2%	Same as above, except less fatigue and depression than with brimonidine 0.2%	Same as above
Carbonic anhydrase inhibitors							
Oral							
Acetazolamide	125 mg	Seldom used for IOP-lowering therapy	Decreases aqueous production	15%–20%	None	Poor tolerance of carbonated beverages, acidosis, depression, malaise, hirsutism, flatulence, paresthesias, numbness, lethargy, blood dyscrasias, diarrhea, weight loss, renal stones, loss of libido, impotence, bone marrow depression, hypokalemia, cramps, anorexia, altered taste, increased serum urate, enuresis	May cause allergic reaction in persons with sulfa allergy Use with caution in patients susceptible to ketoacidosis or hepatic insufficiency Caution for using an oral CAI with other drugs that cause potassium loss Peak: 3–6 hours (sustained release) 2–4 hours (oral)
	250 mg	2–4 times daily					
	500 mg (sustained release)	2 times daily					

Class/Compound	Concentration	Dosing	Mechanism of Action	IOP Reduction	Adverse Effects		Comments, Including Time to Peak Effect and Washout
					Ocular	Systemic	
Acetazolamide (parenteral)	500 mg 5–10 mg/kg	Usually every 6–8 hours	Same as above	Same as above	Same as above	Same as above	Same as above
Methazolamide	25, 50 mg	2–3 times daily	Same as above	Same as above	Same as above	Same as above	Same as above
Topical							
Dorzolamide	2%	2–3 times daily	Same as above	15%–20%	Induced myopia, blurred vision, stinging, keratitis, punctate keratopathy, conjunctivitis, dermatitis	Less likely to induce systemic effects of CAI, but may occur; bitter taste	Peak: 2–3 hours Washout: 48 hours
Brinzolamide	1%	2–3 times daily	Same as above	Same as above	Same as above, except less stinging when compared with dorzolamide	Same as above	Same as above
Parasympathomimetic agents (miotics)							
Cholinergic agonist (direct acting)							
Pilocarpine HCl	0.5, 1.0, 2.0, 3.0, 4.0, 6.0%	2–4 times daily	Increases trabecular outflow	15%–25%	Posterior synechiae, keratitis, miosis, brow ache, cataract growth, angle-closure potential, myopia, retinal tear/detachment, dermatitis, change in retinal sensitivity, color vision changes, epiphora	Increased salivation, increased secretion (gastric), abdominal cramps	Exacerbation of cataract effect; more effective in lighter irides Peak: 1$\frac{1}{2}$–2 hours Washout: 48 hours
Anticholinesterase agent (indirect acting)							
Echothiophate iodide	0.125%	1–2 times daily	Same as above	15%–25%	Intense miosis, iris pigment cyst, myopia, cataract, retinal detachment, angle closure, punctal stenosis, pseudopemphigoid, epiphora	Same as pilocarpine; more gastrointestinal difficulties	Increased inflammation with ocular surgery; may be helpful in aphakia, anesthesia risks (prolonged recovery); useful in eyelid-lash lice, cataract surgery postoperatively

(Continued)

Class/Compound	Concentration	Dosing	Mechanism of Action	IOP Reduction	Ocular	Systemic	Comments, Including Time to Peak Effect and Washout
					Adverse Effects		
Fixed combinations							
Timolol/ brinzolamide	0.5%/1%	2 times daily	Reduces aqueous secretion	25%–30%	Same as those of nonselective β-adrenergic antagonist, topical CAI	Same as those of nonselective β-adrenergic antagonist, topical CAI	—
Timolol/dorzolamide	0.5%/2%	2 times daily	Decreases aqueous production	25%–30%	Same as those of nonselective β-blocker, topical CAI	Same as those of nonselective β-blocker, topical CAI	Peak: 2–3 hours Washout: 1 month
Timolol/latanoprost	0.5%/0.005%	Once daily (nighttime)	Same as nonselective β-blocker and latanoprost	Greater than monotherapy with each individually	Same as those of nonselective β-blocker and latanoprost	Same as those of nonselective β-blocker and latanoprost	Not currently available in the United States
Timolol/travoprost	0.5%/0.004%	Once daily (nighttime)	Same as nonselective β-blocker and travoprost	Same as above	Same as those of nonselective β-blocker and travoprost	Same as nonselective β-blocker and travoprost	Same as above
Timolol/bimatoprost	0.5%/0.03%	Once daily (nighttime)	Same as nonselective β-blocker and bimatoprost	Same as above	Same as those of nonselective β-blocker and bimatoprost	Same as nonselective β-blocker and bimatoprost	Same as above
Timolol/brimonidine tartrate	0.5%/0.2%	2 times daily	Same as nonselective β-blocker and α-agonist	Same as above	Same as those of nonselective β-blocker and α-agonist	Same as those of nonselective β-blocker and α-agonist	—
Brimonidine/ brinzolamide	0.2%/1%	2–3 times daily	Decreases aqueous production; may increase uveoscleral outflow	26%–36%	Same as those of the individual components	Same as those of the individual components	—
Hyperosmotic agents							
Mannitol (parenteral)	20%	0.5–2.0 g/kg body weight	Creates osmotic gradient; dehydrates vitreous	—	IOP rebound, increased aqueous flare	Urinary retention, headache, congestive heart failure, diabetic complications, nausea, vomiting, diarrhea, electrolyte disturbance, confusion, backache, myocardial infarction	Contraindicated in patients in renal failure or on dialysis; caution in heart failure; useful in acute increased IOP
Glyceral (oral)	50%	1–1.5 g/kg	Same as above	—	Similar to above	Similar to above; can cause problems in diabetic patients	Similar to above; may precipitate diabetic ketoacidosis

For an updated version of this table, go to www.aao.org/bcsc_s10_table7-1.

prostaglandin analogue ophthalmic solution available in the United States, appears to be slightly less efficacious than latanoprost (Table 7-2; see also General Approach to Medical Treatment for discussion of preservatives). All of these drugs are used once daily, usually at night, and are less effective when used twice daily. Because some patients may respond better to one agent in this class than to another, switching drugs after a trial of 4–6 weeks may prove helpful.

Adverse Effects

An adverse effect unique to this class of drugs is the darkening of the iris and periocular skin as a result of an increased number of melanosomes within the melanocytes. Increased iris pigmentation is permanent, and the frequency of this effect depends on baseline eye color. Most published data on this increased pigmentation relate to latanoprost and suggest a risk of up to 33% after 5 years of use. In particular, up to 79% of persons with green-brown irides and up to 85% of persons with hazel (yellow-brown) irides may be affected, compared with 8% of persons with blue irides. There are no data to suggest that this color change confers any risk to the patient.

Other adverse effects reported in association with the use of a topical prostaglandin analogue include conjunctival hyperemia (a result of vasodilation and more common with bimatoprost and travoprost), hypertrichosis (Fig 7-1), trichiasis, and distichiasis. These effects appear to be reversible with drug discontinuation.

Table 7-2 Preservative-Free and Alternatively Preserved Ocular Hypotensive Agents

Medication	Preservative
Brimonidine 0.1% (Alphagan P)	Sodium chlorite (Purite)
Dorzolamide-timolol (PF Cosopt)	Preservative-free unit dose vials
Tafluprost	Preservative-free unit dose vials
Timolol	Preservative-free unit dose vials
Timolol gel-forming solution	Benzododecinium bromide (a detergent closely related to BAK)
Travoprost (Travatan Z)	Borate, sorbitol, propylene glycol, and zinc (Sofzia)

BAK = benzalkonium chloride.

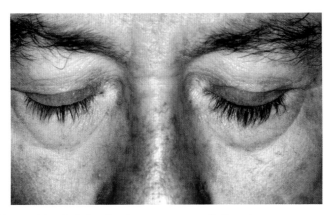

Figure 7-1 Hypertrichosis following latanoprost use (left eye). *(Courtesy of F. Jane Durcan, MD.)*

Use of prostaglandin analogue eyedrops has also been associated with the development of *prostaglandin-associated periorbitopathy*, a complex of periorbital abnormalities that includes deepening of the upper eyelid sulcus, upper eyelid ptosis, enophthalmos, inferior scleral show, and possibly a tight orbit. These abnormalities appear to be the result of periorbital fat atrophy. It is not clear whether this periorbitopathy is reversible.

The development or exacerbation of preexisting cystoid macular edema (CME) can occur in certain predisposed eyes (ie, aphakic eyes, pseudophakic eyes with open posterior capsules, and uveitic eyes). Reactivation of herpetic keratitis can occur. A nongranulomatous anterior uveitis may occur as an idiosyncratic reaction in approximately 1% of patients.

Camras CB, Alm A, Watson P, Stjernschantz J. Latanoprost, a prostaglandin analog, for glaucoma therapy. Efficacy and safety after 1 year of treatment in 198 patients. Latanoprost Study Groups. *Ophthalmology.* 1996;103(11):1916–1924.

Adrenergic Drugs

β-Adrenergic Antagonists

Mechanism of action

Topical β-adrenergic antagonists, or *β-blockers,* lower IOP by inhibiting cyclic adenosine monophosphate (cAMP) production in ciliary epithelium, thereby reducing aqueous humor secretion by 20%–50% (2.5 μL/min to 1.9 μL/min), with a corresponding IOP reduction of 20%–30%. The effect on aqueous production occurs within 1 hour of instillation and can last for up to 4 weeks after discontinuation of the medication. Because systemic absorption occurs, an IOP-lowering effect may also be observed in the untreated contralateral eye. β-Blockers have much less effect on aqueous production during sleep, as aqueous production is already reduced at night; they are thus ineffective in lowering IOP during sleep.

Available agents and dosing frequency

In the United States and Europe, 6 topical β-adrenergic antagonists are approved for the treatment of glaucoma: betaxolol, carteolol, levobunolol, metipranolol, timolol maleate, and timolol hemihydrate. Betaxolol, the only β_1-selective antagonist of the 6 agents, is less effective in lowering IOP than the others, which are nonselective β-adrenergic antagonists. Most β-blockers are approved for twice-daily therapy. In many cases, the nonselective agents can be used once daily. Generally, dosing first thing in the morning is preferred in order to effectively blunt an early-morning pressure rise while minimizing the risk of systemic hypotension during sleep. Many nonselective β-blockers are available in more than one concentration. Clinical experience has shown that in many patients, timolol maleate 0.25% is as effective as timolol maleate 0.5% in lowering IOP.

Approximately 10%–20% of the patients treated with topical β-blockers fail to respond with a significantly lower IOP. Patients already taking a systemic β-blocker may experience little additional IOP lowering from the addition of a topical β-blocker. Extended use of β-blockers may reduce their effectiveness, because the response of β-adrenergic receptors is affected by constant exposure to an agonist (as in long-term drift or tachyphylaxis). Similarly, receptor saturation (drug-induced upregulation of β-adrenergic receptors) may occur within a few weeks of starting these drugs, with loss of effectiveness (eg, short-term escape).

Adverse effects

The ocular and systemic adverse effects of β-adrenergic antagonists are listed in Table 7-1. Plasma drug levels from topical medications can approach those achieved with systemic administration because of the lack of first-pass hepatic metabolism with topical administration and because of their absorption in the nasolacrimal drainage system. However, administering topical medications in a gel vehicle results in reduced systemic absorption and decreased plasma concentrations of β-blockers compared with the equivalent solution.

Systemic adverse effects of β-adrenergic antagonists include bronchospasm, bradycardia, increased heart block, lowered blood pressure, reduced exercise tolerance, and central nervous system (CNS) depression. Patients with diabetes mellitus may experience reduced glucose tolerance and masking of hypoglycemic signs and symptoms. In addition, abrupt withdrawal of ocular β-blockers can exacerbate symptoms of hyperthyroidism.

Before a β-blocker is prescribed, the clinician should ask whether the patient has a history of asthma, as β-blockers may induce severe, life-threatening bronchospasm in susceptible patients. Because betaxolol is a selective β_1 antagonist, it is safer than the nonselective β-blockers for use in patients with asthma; β_2 receptors are present in bronchial smooth muscle cells and their inhibition results in bronchospasm in susceptible individuals. In addition, betaxolol may be less likely to cause depression. However, β-blocker–related adverse effects can still occur.

Prior to initiation of therapy with a topical β-blocker, the patient's pulse should be measured; β-blockers should be withheld if the pulse rate is slow or if more than first-degree heart block is present. Administration of topical β-blockers has been associated with the development of signs and symptoms of myasthenia gravis in patients without a preexisting diagnosis and can exacerbate the condition in patients already known to have the disease. The mechanism by which this occurs is unclear.

Other adverse effects of β-blockers include lethargy, mood changes, depression, altered mentation, light-headedness, syncope, visual disturbance, corneal anesthesia, punctate keratitis, allergy, impotence, reduced libido, and alteration of serum lipids. In children, β-blockers should be used with caution, because of the relatively high systemic levels achieved.

Van Buskirk EM. Adverse reactions from timolol administration. *Ophthalmology.* 1980;87(5): 447–450.

Adrenergic Agonists

The nonselective adrenergic agonists epinephrine (adrenaline) and dipivefrin (a prodrug of epinephrine) reduce aqueous humor production, increase uveoscleral outflow, and improve conventional outflow facility. Both have largely been superseded by other classes of drugs and are now rarely used in the management of glaucoma.

α₂-Selective adrenergic agonists

Mechanism of action α_2-Selective agonists lower IOP by reducing aqueous humor production. The α_2-adrenoceptor found on the ciliary epithelium is coupled to an inhibitory G protein. When this adrenoceptor is bound by catecholamines or pharmacologically active α_2-agonists, it is thought that an intracellular cascade results in reduction in the activity of adenylate cyclase and the intracellular concentration of cAMP, with a resultant reduction in the rate of aqueous humor production. An alternate or possibly complementary mechanism by which aqueous humor production is reduced may be anterior segment vasoconstriction and reduced blood flow to the ciliary body. After a longer period of therapy, increased uveoscleral outflow has also been observed with the selective α_2-adrenergic agonist brimonidine, but not with apraclonidine. How uveoscleral outflow may be increased with brimonidine is unclear, but evidence points to relaxation of ciliary smooth muscle cells. As with β-blockers, systemic absorption of α_2-selective agonists may lead to a crossover effect, although it appears to be small.

Available agents and dosing frequency Brimonidine tartrate is the most commonly used α_2-adrenergic agonist. Apraclonidine hydrochloride (para-aminoclonidine), an α_2-adrenergic agonist and clonidine derivative, is rarely used for long-term therapy because of the frequent occurrence of tachyphylaxis and a hypersensitivity reaction that can cause blepharoconjunctivitis. Apraclonidine is typically used perioperatively to diminish acute IOP spikes that may occur after laser iridotomy, laser trabeculoplasty, Nd:YAG laser capsulotomy, and cataract extraction.

Brimonidine is similarly effective when used perioperatively. In addition, tachyphylaxis is less profound with brimonidine than with apraclonidine. Brimonidine's peak IOP reduction is approximately 26% (2 hours post dose), which is comparable to the reduction achieved by a nonselective β-blocker and superior to that of the selective β-blocker betaxolol. At trough (12 hours post dose), the reduction is only 14%–15%, or less than the reduction achieved with nonselective β-blockers. Studies have shown that brimonidine does not lower nocturnal IOP. Though approved for therapy 3 times daily in the United States, brimonidine is commonly used twice daily, particularly when used in combination with at least one other agent.

Adverse effects The incidence of ocular allergic reactions (eg, follicular conjunctivitis and contact blepharodermatitis; Fig 7-2) is lower with brimonidine than with apracloni-

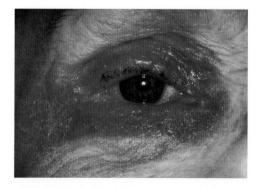

Figure 7-2 Contact blepharodermatitis following α-adrenergic agonist use. *(Courtesy of F. Jane Durcan, MD.)*

dine: less than 15% for brimonidine tartrate 0.2% preserved with benzalkonium chloride, and less than 10% for brimonidine tartrate 0.1% preserved with sodium chlorite (Purite). Cross-sensitivity to brimonidine in patients with known hypersensitivity to apraclonidine is minimal. The incidence of long-term intolerance to brimonidine due to local adverse effects, however, is high (>20%). Granulomatous anterior uveitis is rare but has been reported in association with the use of brimonidine.

α_2-Selective agonists have some α_1-binding activity. The ocular effects of α_1-adrenergic agonists include conjunctival vasoconstriction, pupillary dilation, and eyelid retraction. Apraclonidine has a much greater affinity for α_1-receptors than does brimonidine and is therefore more likely to produce these effects.

Systemic adverse effects of α_2-selective agonists include xerostomia (dry mouth) and lethargy, both mediated by their clonidine-like CNS activity. Brimonidine should not be used in infants and young children because of the risk of CNS depression, apnea, bradycardia, and hypotension, presumably due to increased CNS penetration of the drug.

Monoamine oxidase inhibitors and tricyclic antidepressants may interfere with metabolism of apraclonidine and brimonidine, resulting in toxicity.

Robin AL. Argon laser trabeculoplasty medical therapy to prevent the intraocular pressure rise associated with argon laser trabeculoplasty. *Ophthalmic Surg.* 1991;22(1):31–37.

Schuman JS, Horwitz B, Choplin NT, David R, Albracht D, Chen K. A 1-year study of brimonidine twice daily in glaucoma and ocular hypertension. A controlled, randomized, multicenter clinical trial. Chronic Brimonidine Study Group. *Arch Ophthalmol.* 1997; 115(7):847–852.

Carbonic Anhydrase Inhibitors

Mechanism of Action

Carbonic anhydrase inhibitors (CAIs) decrease aqueous humor production by inhibiting the activity of ciliary epithelial carbonic anhydrase. Systemic CAI therapy may further decrease aqueous humor formation because of the resultant renal metabolic acidosis, which may interfere with activity of ciliary epithelial Na^+,K^+-ATPase. The enzyme carbonic anhydrase is present in many tissues, including corneal endothelium, iris, retinal pigment epithelium, red blood cells, brain, and kidney. More than 90% of the ciliary epithelial enzyme activity must be abolished to decrease aqueous production and lower IOP.

Available Agents and Dosing Frequency

The topical CAI agents, dorzolamide and brinzolamide, are available for long-term treatment of elevated IOP and have fewer systemic adverse effects than the systemic CAIs. In the United States, they are currently approved for use 3 times daily, but most clinicians prescribe them for twice-daily use in many patients. Thrice-daily dosing results in slightly greater IOP reduction. For patients taking an oral CAI, there is no advantage to adding a topical CAI.

Systemic CAIs can be given orally or intravenously and are most useful in acute situations (eg, acute primary angle closure). Oral CAIs begin to act within 1 hour of administration, with maximal effect within 2–4 hours, whereas intravenous CAIs begin to act within 15 minutes. Sustained-release acetazolamide can reach peak effect within 3–6 hours of administration. Because of the adverse effects of systemic CAIs, however, long-term therapy should be reserved for patients whose glaucoma is not controlled with topical therapy and who have refused surgery or in whom surgery would be inappropriate.

The most commonly used oral CAIs are acetazolamide and methazolamide. Compared to acetazolamide, methazolamide has a longer duration of action and is less bound to serum protein; however, it is less effective. Methazolamide and sustained-release acetazolamide are the best tolerated of the systemic CAIs. Methazolamide is metabolized by the liver. Acetazolamide, which is not metabolized, is excreted by the kidney; it must be used with caution and at an adjusted dose in those with renal insufficiency.

Because oral CAIs are potent medications with significant adverse effects (see the following subsection), the lowest dose that reduces the IOP to an acceptable range should be used. Methazolamide is often effective in doses as low as 25–50 mg, given 2 or 3 times daily. Sustained-release formulations of acetazolamide may have fewer adverse effects than its standard formulation. The typical dosage of acetazolamide is 250 mg 4 times a day; for sustained release, it is 500 mg twice a day.

Adverse Effects and Contraindications

Common adverse effects of topical CAIs include bitter taste, blurred vision, burning upon instillation, and punctate keratopathy. Dorzolamide, a solution, may cause burning, as it is formulated at a low pH due to the low solubility of the molecule at physiologic pH levels. Use of brinzolamide, a suspension, results in white deposits in the tear film. Eyes with compromised endothelial cell function may also be at risk of corneal decompensation with use of either of these drugs.

Adverse effects of systemic CAI therapy are usually dose-related and are primarily driven by the resultant metabolic acidosis. Many patients develop paresthesias of the fingers or toes and report loss of energy and anorexia. Weight loss is common. Severe mental depression, abdominal discomfort, diarrhea, loss of libido, impotence, and taste disturbance, especially with carbonated beverages, may also occur. There is a risk of sickle cell crisis in sickle cell anemia and an increased risk of formation of calcium oxalate and calcium phosphate renal stones. Because methazolamide causes less acidosis, it may be less likely than acetazolamide to cause renal lithiasis.

As the urine becomes more alkaline, ammonia excretion is reduced. Systemic CAIs should be avoided in patients with hepatic cirrhosis, as either systemic agent can precipitate hepatic encephalopathy due to increased serum ammonia levels.

CAIs are chemically derived from sulfa drugs and thus may cause an allergic reaction in individuals with sulfa allergies; however, the level of cross-reactivity is low. Aplastic anemia is a rare but potentially fatal idiosyncratic reaction to CAIs. Thrombocytopenia and agranulocytosis can also occur. Although routine complete blood counts have been suggested, they are not predictive of this idiosyncratic reaction and are not routinely recommended. Hypokalemia is a potentially serious complication that is especially likely to occur when an oral CAI is used concurrently with another drug that causes potassium loss (eg, thiazide diuretic). Serum potassium should be checked regularly in such cases.

Fraunfelder FT, Fraunfelder FW, Chambers WA. *Drug-Induced Ocular Side Effects.* 7th ed. Boston: Butterworth-Heinemann; 2014.

Strahlman E, Tipping R, Vogel R. A double-masked, randomized 1-year study comparing dorzolamide (Trusopt), timolol, and betaxolol. International Dorzolamide Study Group. *Arch Ophthalmol.* 1995;113(8):1009–1016.

Parasympathomimetic Agents

Parasympathomimetic agents, or *miotics,* have been used in the treatment of glaucoma for more than 100 years. Traditionally, they are divided into direct-acting cholinergic agonists and indirect-acting anticholinesterase agents. The direct-acting agent pilocarpine continues to be used in certain circumstances, although it is not commonly prescribed for long-term use. In patients with pigmentary glaucoma, pilocarpine is effective in blunting the IOP spike that can occur with jarring physical activities such as running. This drug is also useful in the management of plateau iris syndrome. It has been associated with poor patient adherence to the treatment regimen because of its adverse effect profile and because of its 3 or 4 times-daily dosing; therefore, it is infrequently used. Indirect-acting agents fell out of favor because of their ocular and systemic adverse effects. The indirect-acting agents can be very effective and well tolerated in aphakic eyes with glaucoma, but they are rarely used.

Mechanism of Action

Parasympathomimetics reduce IOP by causing the longitudinal ciliary muscle fibers that insert into the scleral spur and trabecular meshwork to contract, thereby improving outflow facility. Direct-acting agents affect the motor end plates in the same way as acetylcholine, which is transmitted at postganglionic parasympathetic junctions, as well as at other autonomic, somatic, and central synapses. Pilocarpine can reduce IOP by 15%–25%. Indirect-acting agents inhibit the enzyme acetylcholinesterase, thereby prolonging and enhancing the action of naturally secreted acetylcholine. Currently accepted indications for miotic therapy include long-term treatment of elevated IOP in eyes with drainage angles that are persistently occludable despite laser iridotomy (plateau iris syndrome).

Adverse Effects

Miotic agents have been associated with numerous ocular side effects. Induced myopia resulting from ciliary muscle contraction is a side effect of all cholinergic agents; brow ache may accompany the ciliary spasm. The miosis interferes with vision in dim light conditions; in patients with lens opacities, vision is affected in all light conditions. Because miotic agents have been associated with retinal detachment, a peripheral retinal evaluation is suggested before the initiation of therapy. Miotics, particularly the indirect-acting agents, are cataractogenic and may cause iris pigment epithelial cysts and epiphora (a result of direct lacrimal stimulation and punctal stenosis). Ocular surface abnormalities can result in drug-induced pseudopemphigoid. Other potential ocular adverse effects include increased bleeding during surgery and increased inflammation and severe fibrinous iridocyclitis postoperatively. Because miotics can break down the blood–aqueous barrier, they should be avoided in uveitic glaucoma. Occasionally, miotics induce a paradoxical angle closure, particularly in eyes with phacomorphic narrow angles; ciliary muscle contraction leads to forward movement of the lens–iris interface and increased anteroposterior lens diameter, which may cause or exacerbate pupillary block in eyes with a large lens. Systemic adverse effects, seen mainly with indirect-acting medications, include diarrhea, abdominal cramps, increased salivation, bronchospasm, and even enuresis. Depolarizing muscle relaxants such as succinylcholine cannot be used for up to 6 weeks after stopping indirect-acting agents.

Rho Kinase Inhibitors

Two rho kinase inhibitors are approved for clinical use, ripasudil (Japan) and netarsudil (United States). They are thought to lower IOP mainly by relaxing the cytoskeleton of trabecular meshwork and Schlemm canal cells, thereby reducing cell stiffness and increasing conventional outflow facility. Further, netarsudil is a norepinephrine transporter inhibitor and thus is thought to lower episcleral venous pressure. See BCSC Section 2, *Fundamentals and Principles of Ophthalmology,* for further discussion.

Combined Medications

Medications combined in a single bottle have the potential benefits of improved convenience and patient adherence and reduced cost. Fixed combinations consisting of timolol and another agent—a CAI (dorzolamide or brinzolamide), an α_2-adrenergic agonist (brimonidine), or a prostaglandin analogue (latanoprost, travoprost, or bimatoprost)—are available in many countries (see Table 7-1). A fixed combination of brimonidine and brinzolamide is also available. The efficacy of fixed-combination formulations is similar to that of the components instilled separately. With fixed-combination agents that include a β-blocker, the total amount of that agent given may be more than what is needed, as nearly the full effect of a β-blocker can be achieved with once-daily dosing. The ocular side effects are the same as for both drugs given individually. Except in the setting of an acutely elevated or dangerously high IOP, clinicians should make sure each component of the fixed combination is effective in further lowering the IOP by adding the individual components sequentially.

Strohmaier K, Snyder E, DuBiner H, Adamsons I. The efficacy and safety of the dorzolamide-timolol combination versus the concomitant administration of its components. Dorzolamide-Timolol Study Group. *Ophthalmology.* 1998;105(10):1936–1944.

Hyperosmotic Agents

Hyperosmotic agents are used to control acute episodes of elevated IOP. Common hyperosmotic agents include oral glycerol and intravenous mannitol.

When given systemically, hyperosmotic agents increase the blood osmolality, which creates an osmotic gradient between the blood and the vitreous humor, drawing water from the vitreous cavity and reducing IOP. Because of the increased gradient, the larger the dose administered and the more rapid the administration, the greater the subsequent IOP reduction. A substance distributed only in extracellular water (eg, mannitol), is more effective than a drug distributed in total body water (eg, urea). The osmotic agent enters the eye faster when the blood–aqueous barrier is disrupted than when it is intact, reducing the effectiveness of the drug and its duration of action.

Hyperosmotic agents are rarely administered for longer than a few hours because their effects are transient (a result of the rapid reequilibration of the osmotic gradient). They become less effective over time, and a rebound elevation in IOP may occur if the agent penetrates the eye and reverses the osmotic gradient.

Adverse effects of these drugs include headache, confusion, backache, acute congestive heart failure, and myocardial infarction. The rapid increase in extracellular volume and cardiac preload caused by hyperosmotic agents may precipitate or aggravate congestive heart failure. Intravenous administration is more likely to cause this problem than oral administration. In addition, subdural and subarachnoid hemorrhages have been reported after treatment with hyperosmotic agents. Glycerol can precipitate hyperglycemia or even ketoacidosis in patients with diabetes mellitus, because it is metabolized into sugar and ketone bodies. Like oral CAIs, hyperosmotics are contraindicated in patients in renal failure or on dialysis.

General Approach to Medical Treatment

Long-Term Therapy

The ophthalmologist should tailor therapy for open-angle glaucoma to the individual needs of the patient, including establishing a target IOP. Though important, IOP is only one of several factors to monitor. The effectiveness of the therapy can be determined only by careful, repeated scrutiny of the patient's optic nerve, retinal nerve fiber layer, and visual field status (see Chapter 3).

As mentioned, characteristics of the medical agents available for the treatment of glaucoma are summarized in Table 7-1. When making management decisions, ophthalmologists should keep in mind the efficacy, side effect profile, and cost of the drug, as well as the likelihood of patient adherence to the drug regimen. Treatment is usually initiated with a single topical medication, unless the baseline IOP is extremely high, in which case 2 or more medications may be indicated. A discussion with the patient regarding treatment options can be beneficial for determining the optimal choice.

Prostaglandin analogues, β-blockers, α_2-adrenergic agonists, and topical CAIs are all reasonable choices as first-line therapy for open-angle glaucoma, as is laser trabeculoplasty; however, prostaglandin analogues are the most commonly utilized because of their superior efficacy, once-daily dosing, and favorable safety profile. Although the local adverse effects of β-blockers are minimal, the potential systemic adverse effects of these drugs are significant and they lack nocturnal IOP-lowering efficacy.

If one agent is not adequate to reduce the IOP to the desired range, the initial agent may be discontinued and another tried. If no single agent controls the pressure, a combination of topical agents should be used. Again, customizing the choice of agent to the patient's needs is helpful when selecting additional medication(s). In unusual circumstances, this might include miotic therapy for patients with aphakia and, in some instances, systemic CAIs for short periods when the clinical situation warrants the risk of adverse effects associated with CAI use. Clearly, when 3 or more medications are required, patient adherence to the medication regimen becomes more difficult and the potential for local and systemic adverse effects increases. Laser trabeculoplasty is a reasonable choice for initial or add-on therapy (see Chapter 8 for more information on this procedure). Further, patients may not be able to tolerate multiple topical agents because of preservative toxicity. Benzalkonium chloride (BAK), the agent most commonly used as a preservative, is present in most of the currently available topical ophthalmic eyedrops. If a reaction is suspected, an ocular hypotensive agent with an alternative preservative or preservative-free formulation can be used (see Table 7-2).

For rehabilitation of the ocular surface, it may be beneficial to stop all topical medications—if the level of glaucomatous damage permits—and have the patient use preservative-free artificial tears frequently. During this period, the temporary use of oral CAIs may be helpful to lower IOP, if clinically warranted.

Patients sometimes fail to associate systemic adverse effects with topical drugs and, consequently, seldom volunteer symptoms. The ophthalmologist must make sure to inquire about these symptoms. In addition, communicating with the primary care physician is important not only to provide information about the potential adverse effects of glaucoma medication but also to discuss the effects that other currently prescribed medications (eg, for systemic disease) might have on the glaucomatous process. Modification of oral β-blocker therapy for hypertension, for example, may affect IOP.

Therapy for Acute Intraocular Pressure Elevation

The goal of medical treatment of acute IOP elevation is usually lowering IOP in order to prevent further damage to the optic nerve; clearing the cornea of edema, if present; and reducing intraocular inflammation. Hyperosmotic agents and systemic CAIs may be required in order to lower the IOP in eyes with acute IOP elevation prior to definitive treatment. In the case of acute primary angle closure, lowering the IOP also facilitates pupillary constriction before an iridotomy is performed (see Chapter 5).

Administration of Ocular Medications

Patients should be shown how to instill eyedrops properly and should be given instruction on nasolacrimal occlusion, which can be used to reduce the systemic absorption of topical ocular medications and to prolong their ocular contact time. Directing the patient to close the eyes for 1–3 minutes after instillation of the eyedrop will also promote corneal penetration and reduce systemic absorption of the drug by reducing the flow of medication-containing tears into the nasolacrimal drainage system.

Proper instillation procedures are especially important with the use of β-blockers, α_2-adrenergic agonists, and topical CAIs (to minimize the likelihood of taste disturbance). In addition, these procedures ensure that there is a sufficient amount of time between the instillation of different medications; eyedrops that need to be administered at the same time should be separated by at least 5 minutes to prevent washout of the first drug by the second. Patients should be taught how to space their medications, and instructional charts should be given. A dosing aid device may also be considered, especially for patients who live alone or who are unable to successfully instill eyedrops.

Use of Glaucoma Medications During Pregnancy or by Breastfeeding Mothers

Often, IOP decreases during pregnancy, both in healthy subjects and in patients with glaucoma. However, glaucoma patients who are pregnant frequently continue to require ocular hypotensive medical therapy throughout the pregnancy. As mentioned previously, topical ocular hypotensive medications are systemically absorbed; they subsequently cross the placenta and enter the fetal circulation or can be secreted into breast milk.

Unfortunately, there is little definitive information concerning the safety of glaucoma medication use in pregnant women or breastfeeding mothers. In the US Food and Drug Administration (FDA) drug classification system, the rating *Pregnancy Category B* indicates that animal studies of the drug have revealed no harm to the fetus, but no adequate and well-controlled studies have been done in pregnant women; or, animal studies of this drug have shown an adverse effect, but adequate and well-controlled studies in pregnant woman have failed to demonstrate a risk to the fetus. The *Pregnancy Category C* rating indicates that no animal studies have been conducted and that it is not known whether the drug can cause harm when given to a pregnant woman. The drug should be used during pregnancy only if clearly indicated. This category also includes drugs that have shown an adverse effect in animal studies, but there are no adequate and well-controlled studies of these drugs in pregnant women. Brimonidine is the only glaucoma agent with a Pregnancy Category B rating; all other agents have a Pregnancy Category C rating.

There are reports of growth retardation, arrhythmia, bradycardia, and lethargy affecting the fetus or newborn exposed to β-adrenergic antagonists. These agents are concentrated in breast milk and should be avoided in breastfeeding mothers because of their potential adverse effects on infants. If a β-adrenergic antagonist must be used during pregnancy or during breastfeeding, the fetus or infant must be carefully monitored and the lowest effective dose should be utilized.

Brimonidine, though reasonably safe to use during pregnancy, has been reported to cause apnea in infants and young children and should not be used in these patients. Brimonidine should be discontinued prior to delivery to minimize the risk of this complication in the newborn.

The CAIs have been shown to be teratogenic in rodents. Systemic CAIs should be avoided during pregnancy, and it is preferable to avoid the use of topical CAIs in pregnant women, if possible.

Because prostaglandins increase uterine contractility and may induce labor, albeit when given at much higher doses than those used in topical therapy, there is a theoretical risk to the pregnancy. With all topical ocular hypotensive medications, pregnant and breastfeeding patients should be advised to perform nasolacrimal occlusion during eyedrop instillation. In general, it is prudent to minimize the use of medications in pregnant women whenever possible. The clinician may want to consider laser trabeculoplasty or other surgical intervention in cases in which the benefits outweigh the potential risks.

Brauner SC, Chen TC, Hutchinson BT, Chang MA, Pasquale LR, Grosskreutz CL. The course of glaucoma during pregnancy: a retrospective case series. *Arch Ophthalmol.* 2006;124(8):1089–1094.

Sheth BP. Drugs and pregnancy. *Focal Points: Clinical Modules for Ophthalmologists.* San Francisco: American Academy of Ophthalmology; 2007, module 7.

Use of Glaucoma Medications in Elderly Patients

There are specific considerations regarding the use of glaucoma medications in elderly patients. First, elderly patients generally have greater difficulty instilling their medications than do younger patients; consequently, their adherence to the treatment regimen may be affected. Instillation difficulties may be due to tremor, poor coordination, or a comorbidity such as arthritis. Adherence will also be affected in an elderly patient with reduced mental capacity or poor memory and a complicated drug regimen, especially because this individual is most likely already taking multiple systemic medications for other ailments. Second, elderly persons have a greater susceptibility to the systemic adverse effects of glaucoma medications. The incidence and severity of systemic adverse effects may be higher with β-blockers and α_2-adrenergic agonists in these patients. For example, it has been shown that a significant proportion of asymptomatic elderly patients suffer a significant, but reversible, reduction in pulmonary function with the use of β-blockers.

Diggory P, Cassels-Brown A, Vail A, Abbey LM, Hillman JS. Avoiding unsuspected respiratory side-effects of topical timolol with cardioselective or sympathomimetic agents. *Lancet.* 1995; 345(8965):1604–1606.

Generic Medications

Many glaucoma medications are available as generic drugs. Although the generic agents are required to be chemically or biologically equivalent to the brand-name product, in some cases there may be differences in formulation that could potentially alter a drug's effect. The use of lower-cost generic medications has been shown to improve patient adherence to medication regimens.

Patient Adherence to a Medication Regimen

Glaucoma medications are effective only if patients use them. The first step in improving patient adherence to a medication regimen is patient education. If patients understand the disease and the nature and benefits of treatment, adherence is increased; it is also enhanced when patients are aware of the possible adverse effects of a medication. Patient education should include a discussion of treatment alternatives.

The ophthalmologist must make sure that the patient understands the treatment regimen. Simpler medication regimens can improve patient adherence. The fewest number of medications, instilled with the least frequency, is optimal. If the patient requires multiple medications and doses, it may be helpful to coordinate administration with daily events, such as meals or brushing teeth. A written schedule for medications can also be very helpful. Finally, as mentioned previously, proper instillation of eyedrops, by the patient or someone else, is essential and should be confirmed by the ophthalmologist.

CHAPTER 8

Surgical Therapy for Glaucoma

▶ *This chapter includes related videos, which can be accessed by scanning the QR codes provided in the text or going to www.aao.org/bcscvideo_section10.*

Surgical treatment for glaucoma is usually undertaken when medical therapy is not appropriate, not tolerated, not effective, or not properly used by a particular patient, and the glaucoma remains uncontrolled with either documented progressive damage or a high risk of further damage. Surgery encompasses both laser and incisional procedures.

Laser surgery is used as primary, adjunctive, or prophylactic treatment in various types of glaucoma. For primary angle closure, the most frequent surgeries are laser iridotomy and laser iridoplasty to widen the angle and, less commonly, laser trabeculoplasty and cyclodestruction to lower intraocular pressure (IOP). In open-angle glaucoma, laser trabeculoplasty is most frequently used to lower IOP, but cyclodestruction can also be used in select cases.

Incisional surgery is the first-line treatment for primary congenital glaucoma. For most other types of glaucoma, a trial of medication and/or laser surgery is first attempted to control IOP. The clinician must exercise caution when recommending incisional surgery because potential adverse effects (infections, hypotony, cataracts) can result in vision loss. Early studies of trabeculectomy as initial therapy for glaucoma, which were performed before the introduction of contemporary glaucoma medications, suggested that trabeculectomy might offer some advantages—better control of IOP, reduction in the number of patient visits to the physician, and possibly better preservation of the visual field, for example. The results of the Collaborative Initial Glaucoma Treatment Study (CIGTS; see Chapter 4) confirmed that initial surgical therapy achieves better IOP control than does initial medical therapy. However, this finding did not translate to better visual field stabilization on average because subjects who received initial surgical treatment had a higher risk of cataract in the long term. In both groups, there was a low incidence of visual field progression. However, the 9-year follow-up data showed that initial surgery led to less visual field progression than did initial medical therapy in subjects with advanced visual field loss at baseline, whereas subjects with diabetes mellitus had more visual field loss over time if treated initially with surgery. Based on the results of this study and on current practice, most clinicians defer incisional surgery for primary open-angle glaucoma (POAG) unless initial treatment with medical and/or laser therapy fails. Surgical treatment can be accelerated in patients with advanced visual field loss at presentation.

When surgery is indicated, the clinical setting must guide selection of the appropriate procedure. Each of the many possible procedures is appropriate in specific conditions and clinical situations.

Migdal C, Gregory W, Hitchings R. Long-term functional outcome after early surgery compared with laser and medicine in open-angle glaucoma. *Ophthalmology.* 1994;101(10): 1651–1657.

Musch DC, Gillespie BW, Lichter PR, Niziol LM, Janz NK; CIGTS Study Investigators. Visual field progression in the Collaborative Initial Glaucoma Treatment Study the impact of treatment and other baseline factors. *Ophthalmology.* 2009;116(2):200–207.

Laser Surgery

Laser Trabeculoplasty

Laser trabeculoplasty (LTP) involves application of laser energy to the trabecular meshwork in discrete spots, usually covering 180°–360° per treatment. The goal of LTP is to increase outflow facility and thus reduce IOP. Different laser wavelengths and delivery systems can be used, including argon laser, diode laser, and Q-switched Nd:YAG laser.

The Glaucoma Laser Trial (GLT) was a multicenter randomized clinical trial that assessed the efficacy and safety of argon laser trabeculoplasty (ALT) as an alternative to topical medical therapy in patients with newly diagnosed, previously untreated POAG. The study was flawed in that one eye was assigned to ALT and the fellow eye was assigned to timolol treatment, which can have an effect on the contralateral ALT eye and confound the study results. Within the first 2 years of follow-up, ALT as initial therapy appeared to be as effective as medication. However, more than half of the eyes treated initially with laser required the addition of one or more medications to control IOP over the course of the study.

Mechanism

Several mechanisms of action were initially proposed for the increased outflow facility that occurs following successful LTP. In ALT specifically, thermal damage to the treated trabecular meshwork causes shrinkage of collagen fibers and therefore stretching and widening of adjacent areas to allow for more outflow. In all forms of LTP, most investigators believe that chemical mediators, specifically interleukin-1β and tumor necrosis factor-α, are released from treated trabecular meshwork cells, increasing outflow facility through induction of specific matrix metalloproteinases. The energy of the frequency-doubled Q-switched Nd:YAG laser used in selective laser trabeculoplasty (SLT) is selectively absorbed by pigmented trabecular cells, sparing adjacent cells and tissue from thermal damage. The number of monocytes and macrophages in the trabecular meshwork increases substantially after SLT, and this increase may play a role in lowering IOP.

Kramer TR, Noecker RJ. Comparison of the morphologic changes after selective laser trabeculoplasty and argon laser trabeculoplasty in human eye bank eyes. *Ophthalmology.* 2001;108(4):773–779.

Indications

Many clinicians use medical therapy before advancing to LTP, but LTP is a reasonable initial step in the management of glaucoma and ocular hypertension (discussed in Chapter 4). In addition, patients who cannot tolerate or adhere to initial medical therapy may be candidates for LTP.

Multiple prospective studies have demonstrated that ALT and SLT achieve similar pressure lowering. The IOP-lowering effect of LTP is similar to that of prostaglandin analogues, with LTP expected to lower IOP by 20%–25%. LTP effectively reduces IOP in POAG, pigmentary glaucoma, pseudoexfoliation syndrome, and corticosteroid-induced glaucoma. Aphakic and pseudophakic eyes may respond to LTP less favorably than phakic eyes. IOP control is unlikely to be diminished by subsequent cataract extraction. LTP is not effective for treating certain types of secondary glaucoma, such as uveitic glaucoma.

Contraindications

LTP is not advised in patients with inflammatory glaucoma, iridocorneal endothelial syndrome, neovascular glaucoma, synechial angle closure, or developmental glaucoma. LTP can be tried in angle recession, but the underlying tissue alterations may cause the procedure to be ineffective. Another relative contraindication for LTP is the lack of effect in the fellow eye. If an eye has advanced damage and high IOP, LTP is unlikely to achieve the target pressure (see Chapter 7 for discussion of target pressure).

Preoperative evaluation

As with all ocular surgery, the preoperative evaluation recommended for LTP includes a detailed medical and ocular history and a comprehensive eye examination. Particular attention must be paid to visual field examination, gonioscopy, and optic nerve evaluation; the trabecular meshwork must be visible on gonioscopy. The degree of pigmentation in the angle determines the power setting: the more pigmented the trabecular meshwork, the less energy required.

Technique

In ALT, a 50-μm laser beam of 0.1-second duration is focused through a goniolens at the junction of the anterior nonpigmented and the posterior pigmented edge of the trabecular meshwork (Fig 8-1). Application to the posterior trabecular meshwork tends to result in inflammation, pigment dispersion, prolonged IOP elevation, and peripheral anterior synechiae (PAS) formation. The power setting (300–1000 mW) should be titrated to achieve the desired endpoint, which is blanching of the trabecular meshwork or production of a tiny bubble. If a large bubble appears, the power is reduced and titrated to achieve the proper effect. As LTP was originally described, laser energy was applied to the entire circumference (360°) of the trabecular meshwork. But evidence suggests that a satisfactory reduction in IOP is achieved in many eyes and there is a lower risk of short-term pressure elevation when only half of the circumference is treated, with approximately 40–50 applications over 180° of the meshwork.

The procedure with the diode laser is similar: a 50–75-μm laser beam is focused through a goniolens with a power setting of 600–1000 mW and duration of 0.1 second.

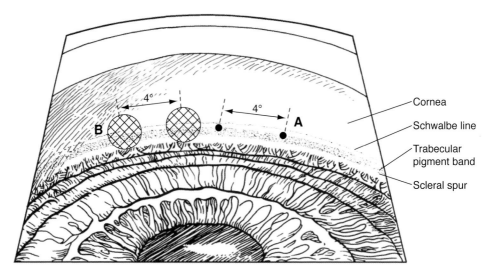

Figure 8-1 Illustration showing the position of argon laser trabeculoplasty *(A)* and selective laser trabeculoplasty *(B)* treatment in the trabecular meshwork.

In SLT, the laser targets intracellular melanin. A frequency-doubled (532-nm) Q-switched Nd:YAG laser with a fixed 400-μm spot size is used to deliver 0.4–1.5 mJ of energy per spot for 3.0 ns, titrated to the appearance of bubbles. Results of clinical studies suggest that the procedure is safe and effective, with IOP-lowering effects similar to those achieved with ALT. Histologic studies have shown that treatment with SLT causes less coagulative damage to and fewer structural changes in the trabecular meshwork compared with treatment with ALT.

Latina MA, Sibayan SA, Shin DH, Noecker RJ, Marcellino G. Q-switched 532-nm Nd:YAG laser trabeculoplasty (selective laser trabeculoplasty): a multicenter, pilot, clinical study. *Ophthalmology.* 1998;105(11):2082–2090.

Complications

The most common complication of LTP is a transient rise in IOP, which occurs in approximately 20% of patients. IOP has been reported to reach 50–60 mm Hg, and this transient rise may cause additional damage to the optic nerve and visual field. This rise is less common when only 180° of the angle is treated per session.

IOP elevations are of particular concern in patients with advanced glaucoma. Rises in IOP are usually evident by the first hour postoperatively. The adjunctive use of topical apraclonidine or brimonidine has been shown to blunt postoperative pressure elevation. Other medications shown to blunt these IOP spikes include β-blockers, pilocarpine, and carbonic anhydrase inhibitors (CAIs). Hyperosmotic agents and oral CAIs may be helpful in eyes with IOP spikes not responsive to topical medications.

Low-grade anterior uveitis may follow LTP. Some surgeons routinely prescribe a course of topical anti-inflammatory drugs for 4–7 days after LTP; others use them only if inflammation develops. PAS may occur after ALT. Other rare complications of LTP include hyphema, corneal inflammation and edema (similar to the diffuse lamellar keratitis seen after corneal refractive surgery), reactivation of herpes simplex virus, and persistently elevated IOP requiring incisional surgery.

Results and long-term follow-up

For follow-up, the surgeon should allow 4–6 weeks before evaluating the full effect of treatment and deciding whether additional treatment is necessary. Approximately 80% of patients with medically uncontrolled open-angle glaucoma experience a drop in IOP for a minimum of 6–12 months following LTP. Longer-term data have shown that 50% of patients with an initial response maintain a significantly lower IOP level for 3–5 years after treatment. The success rate at 10 years is approximately 30%. The highest success rates are seen in older patients with POAG and in pseudoexfoliation glaucoma. Eyes with pigmentary glaucoma may show a good initial decrease in IOP, but with continued pigment shedding, this may not be sustained.

Elevation of IOP may recur in some patients after months or even years of control. Additional laser treatment may be helpful in some patients, especially if the entire angle has not been treated previously. Re-treatment of an angle that has been fully treated (approximately 80–100 applications over 360°) has a lower success rate and a higher complication rate than does primary treatment. Also, the effect after re-treatment may not be as long lasting as that of the first treatment.

Wang W, He M, Zhou M, Zhang X. Selective laser trabeculoplasty versus argon laser trabeculoplasty in patients with open-angle glaucoma: a systematic review and meta-analysis. *PLoS One.* 2013;8(12):e84270.

Wise JB, Witter SL. Argon laser therapy for open-angle glaucoma. A pilot study. *Arch Ophthalmol.* 1979;97(2):319–322.

Laser Iridotomy

Indications

Iridotomy is performed for pupillary block resulting in primary angle closure (PAC) or acute PAC (see Chapter 5). For the PAC suspect (PACS), the use of iridotomy varies widely; experts disagree on the threshold indications at which an iridotomy should be performed. Iridotomy provides an alternate route for aqueous trapped in the posterior chamber to enter the anterior chamber, which then allows the iris to recede from its occlusion of the trabecular meshwork (Fig 8-2). Sometimes it is necessary to perform iridotomy for diagnostic purposes. For example, the diagnosis of plateau iris syndrome is confirmed only when a patent iridotomy fails to change the peripheral iris configuration and relieve angle closure.

Contraindications

A laser iridotomy is not recommended in the case of a completely flat anterior chamber because of the risk of corneal endothelial damage. An opacified or edematous cornea precludes an adequate view. Once 360° of synechial angle closure has occurred, iridotomy offers no benefit. Angle closure from mechanisms other than pupillary block also does not require iridotomy (ie, neovascular glaucoma and iridocorneal endothelial syndrome). An eye with active rubeosis iridis may bleed and develop a large hyphema following laser iridotomy. The risk of bleeding is also increased in a patient taking systemic anticoagulants,

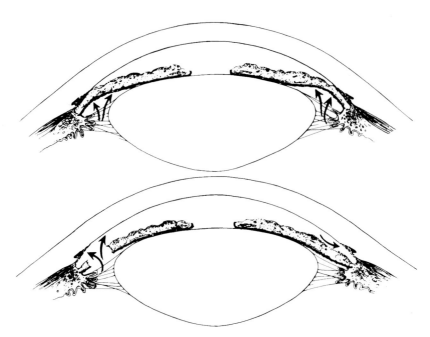

Figure 8-2 Angle-closure glaucoma *(top).* Laser iridotomy or surgical iridectomy breaks the pupillary block and results in opening of the entire peripheral angle *(bottom)* if no permanent peripheral anterior synechiae are present. *(Reproduced and modified with permission from Kolker AE, Hetherington J, eds.* Becker-Shaffer's Diagnosis and Therapy of the Glaucomas. *5th ed. St Louis: Mosby; 1983.)*

including aspirin. The risk of hyphema can be reduced by pretreating dark irides with an argon or diode laser prior to penetration with Nd:YAG laser and/or by coagulating an actively bleeding blood vessel with argon or diode laser.

Preoperative considerations

In acute angle closure, performing laser iridotomy is often difficult due to the cloudy cornea, shallow chamber, and engorged iris that are present in this condition. Before proceeding to surgery, the clinician should attempt to acutely lower the IOP medically with topical medications, intravenous CAIs, or osmotics, which will help clear the cornea and make the patient more comfortable. In some countries, the IOP is initially lowered with a careful paracentesis in addition to medication. Corneal edema may be improved prior to laser iridotomy by pretreatment with topical glycerin. In prophylactic iridotomies, pretreatment with pilocarpine may be helpful by stretching and thinning the iris. Pretreatment with apraclonidine or brimonidine can help blunt IOP spikes. The patient should be asked about anticoagulants, as their use increases the risk of hyphema.

Technique

Laser iridotomies can be performed with the Nd:YAG laser, argon laser, diode laser, or a combination of diode/Nd:YAG or argon/Nd:YAG lasers. For the combined procedure, the argon or diode laser is used first to thin iris tissue and coagulate underlying blood vessels, and then the Nd:YAG laser is used to penetrate the iris. Typical settings for the argon pretreatment are 0.1 seconds, 50-μm spot size, and 900 mW, while the Nd:YAG settings are 2–5 mJ. The surgeon should plan to place the iridotomy in the far periphery of the superior iris, where it will be covered by eyelid, if possible, or at the 3- or 9-o'clock position, to decrease the chances of linear dysphotopsias. It is easiest to penetrate the iris through a crypt.

Nd:YAG iridotomy alone is preferred for many eyes. In general, fewer pulses and less energy is needed to create a patent iridotomy with the Nd:YAG laser alone than with an argon-alone laser peripheral iridotomy (LPI). Also, the effectiveness of the Nd:YAG laser is not affected by iris color, and the iridotomy created by this laser does not close as often over the long term as one created by argon laser. With a condensing contact lens, the typical initial setting for the Nd:YAG laser is 2–8 mJ. Potential complications include disruption of the anterior lens capsule or corneal endothelium, bleeding (usually transient), postoperative spike in IOP, inflammation, and delayed closure of the iridotomy. To prevent damage to the lens, the surgeon must use caution with the Nd:YAG laser when further enlarging the opening once patency has been established.

The argon laser alone can be used for performing iridotomy in most eyes, but very dark and very light irides present technical challenges. With an LPI-specific condensing contact lens in place, the procedure is done in 2 steps: the first step contracts tissue, and the second penetrates it. The typical initial argon laser settings are 0.2–0.5 seconds of duration, 200–500-μm spot size, and 200–400 mW for up to 5 shots; the subsequent laser settings are 0.1 second of duration, 50-μm spot size, and 800–1000 mW for up to 300 shots. There are variations in technique, and iris color dictates which technique is chosen. Complications include localized lens opacity, acute rise in IOP (which may damage the optic nerve), transient or persistent anterior uveitis, early closure of the iridotomy, posterior synechiae, and corneal and retinal burns.

Postoperative care

Bleeding may occur from the iridotomy site, particularly with use of the Nd:YAG laser. Often, compression of the eye with the laser lens will provide a tamponade for the vessel, thereby slowing bleeding until coagulation can occur. In rare cases when this does not work, it may be helpful to use an argon laser to coagulate the vessel. If postoperative spikes in IOP occur, as with LTP, they are treated as described in the section Laser Trabeculoplasty. Topical corticosteroids are usually prescribed for 1 week, longer if necessary, as prophylaxis against inflammation.

Hoskins HD, Migliazzo CV. Laser iridectomy—a technique for blue irises. *Ophthalmic Surg.* 1984;15(6):488–490.

Spaeth GL, Idowu O, Seligsohn A, et al. The effects of iridotomy size and position on symptoms following laser peripheral iridotomy. *J Glaucoma.* 2005;14(5):364–367.

Vera V, Naqi A, Belovay GW, Varma DK, Ahmed Il. Dysphotopsia after temporal versus superior laser peripheral iridotomy: a prospective randomized paired eye trial. *Am J Ophthalmol.* 2014;157(5):929–935.

Laser Gonioplasty, or Peripheral Iridoplasty

Indications

Gonioplasty, or iridoplasty, is a technique to deepen the angle. It is primarily used in persistent appositional angle-closure glaucoma after successful iridotomy in cases of plateau iris syndrome, nanophthalmos, and lens-related angle-closure. It is also used in cases of acute angle closure in which a shallow chamber precludes iridotomy. Stromal burns are made in the peripheral iris with the argon laser to cause contraction and flattening, thereby pulling the iris away from the angle.

Contraindications

The contraindications for gonioplasty are similar to those for laser iridotomy but also include tumors of the iris or ciliary body and uveitis.

Preoperative considerations

An angle that is appositionally closed from plateau iris syndrome will not open after laser iridotomy because forward displacement of the ciliary processes pushes the peripheral iris into the drainage angle.

Technique

Long duration and large spot size with relatively low power is necessary to cause a contraction burn that will thin peripheral iris and pull it out of the angle. Pilocarpine is given preoperatively to maximally stretch the iris, and a contact lens with a gonioscopy mirror is placed on the eye. Typical laser settings for the argon green laser are 0.5 second of duration, 200–500-μm spot size, and 200–400 mW of power. The time and energy can be titrated based on immediate response.

Ritch R, Tham CC, Lam DS. Argon laser peripheral iridoplasty (ALPI): an update. *Surv Ophthalmol.* 2007;52(3):279–288.

Postoperative considerations

Elevated IOP may occur in the postoperative period and should be monitored, as is done after other laser procedures. Anisocoria, iris pigment changes, and corneal endothelial damage can occur. Postoperative anterior uveitis is common and should be treated with topical corticosteroids.

Cyclodestruction

Several surgical procedures reduce aqueous secretion and thus decrease IOP by destroying a portion of the ciliary body. Cyclocryotherapy, thermal lasers, such as continuous-wave Nd:YAG, argon, and diode lasers (Fig 8-3), have been used to inhibit the secretory activity of the ciliary epithelium. Cyclocryotherapy, in which the ciliary body is frozen, and Nd:YAG cyclodestruction were associated with high rates of hypotony and phthisis bulbi. The most common modalities in current practice are endoscopic cyclophotocoagulation and diode laser transscleral cyclophotocoagulation. *Endoscopic cyclophotocoagulation* is an intraocular procedure in which a microendoscope applies laser energy to the ciliary processes under direct visualization. In *transscleral cyclophotocoagulation,* the laser probe is placed externally, which focuses the beam across the sclera to cause destruction of the underlying ciliary body and ciliary epithelium. The risk of hypotony and phthisis bulbi is much lower with these latter modalities (unless the eyes are ischemic), and these modalities have been safely used in eyes with good vision.

Indications

Traditionally, cyclodestruction has been used to lower IOP in eyes that have poor visual potential or that are poor candidates for incisional outflow surgery. The procedure is

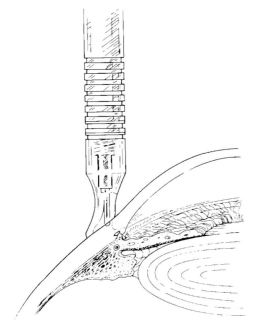

Figure 8-3 Cyclodestruction. The diode laser handpiece attachment from one manufacturer is shown aligned with the limbus and ready to treat. *(Reproduced with permission from Weinreb RN, Mills RP, eds.* Glaucoma Surgery: Principles and Techniques. *2nd ed. Ophthalmology Monograph 4. San Francisco: American Academy of Ophthalmology; 1998:165.)*

useful in all types of glaucoma, and it can be considered for elderly patients when other glaucoma surgeries are refused or not possible because of poor systemic health. Diode laser transscleral cyclodestruction is used by some clinicians for lowering the IOP in painful blind eyes (no light perception) or in eyes that have exhausted outflow procedures. Other interventions available for blind eyes are retrobulbar alcohol injection, retrobulbar chlorpromazine injection, or enucleation. Endoscopic cyclodestruction is used in eyes with better visual potential because there is less damage to the ciliary body.

Contraindications

External cyclodestruction is relatively contraindicated in eyes with good vision because of a moderately high rate of phthisis bulbi and hypotony reported in the literature, although these risks are highest in eyes with a history of neovascular glaucoma. There is also the risk of loss of visual acuity from macular edema. Endoscopic cyclodestruction, an incisional surgery, is contraindicated in blind eyes because of the small risk of sympathetic ophthalmia.

Preoperative considerations

The preoperative evaluation for cyclodestructive procedures is the same as that for incisional glaucoma surgery. Many surgeons choose to perform transscleral cyclodestruction with sedation to make the patient comfortable during the sub-Tenon, peribulbar or retrobulbar block, although the block and transscleral cyclodestruction can be performed in a nonsterile setting without sedation. Endoscopic cyclodestruction requires a sterile operating room because it is an intraocular procedure.

Techniques

Diode laser transscleral cyclophotocoagulation and endoscopic cyclophotocoagulation are replacing cyclocryotherapy and Nd:YAG cyclodestruction, as they are better tolerated and cause less pain and inflammation. Although there is a degree of unpredictability with diode laser cyclodestruction, this method is considerably more predictable in effect than its predecessors.

In transscleral cyclodestruction, the patient is given a local block for anesthesia. The laser energy is delivered via a probe placed on the sclera over the pars plicata. Transillumination should be used if the anatomy is distorted, as in buphthalmic eyes. Each laser application is of long duration (2–4 seconds) and the energy varies (750–2000 mW) depending on the pigmentation of the eye. If tissue disruption is heard via a popping noise, energy should be lowered. The number of applications varies (14–24 on average) and spans 180°–360°. One should avoid the 3- and 9-o'clock positions where the ciliary nerves enter the eye.

In endoscopic cyclodestruction, a sterile surgical field is required, along with a local block for anesthesia. A clear cornea or pars plana incision with vitrectomy is made to accommodate the probe, which is simultaneously used to visualize and treat the ciliary processes until they shrink and turn white. The laser energy is continuous and constant, as long as the probe is held the same distance from the processes. A phakic eye is a relative contraindication to the endoscopic approach.

Postoperative management

Pain after external cyclodestruction may be substantial. Patients should receive adequate analgesics, including narcotics, during the immediate postoperative period. Cycloplegics, corticosteroids, and nonsteroidal anti-inflammatory agents are prescribed for discomfort and inflammation and tapered as the clinical picture allows. IOP-lowering drops are continued until the IOP-lowering effect of cyclodestruction is observed.

Complications

Cyclodestructive procedures may result in prolonged hypotony, pain, inflammation, cystoid macular edema, hemorrhage, retinal detachment, and even phthisis bulbi. Sympathetic ophthalmia is a rare but serious complication. Endophthalmitis is a risk with the endoscopic approach.

Ishida K. Update on results and complications of cyclophotocoagulation. *Curr Opin Ophthalmol.* 2013;24(2):102–110.

Pastor SA, Singh K, Lee DA, et al. Cyclophotocoagulation: a report by the American Academy of Ophthalmology. *Ophthalmology.* 2001;108(11):2130–2138.

Incisional Surgery

The most frequently performed incisional surgeries for glaucoma are trabeculectomy and implantation of tube shunts. These procedures can decrease IOP significantly because they create a pathway that bypasses the eye's natural outflow pathways, but they also carry significant risk of complications. They are the procedures of choice for moderate to severe cases of open-angle and angle-closure glaucoma. There are several procedures that allow for nonpenetrating and/or minimally invasive surgery. These procedures enhance the eye's natural outflow pathway and have a better safety profile than trabeculectomy and tube shunts. However, they tend to lower IOP less effectively. The nonpenetrating and minimally invasive surgeries are used to treat open-angle glaucoma at an earl Cataract surgery alone can decrease IOP in certain eyes, particularly those with high associated with narrow angles from a large lens.

Trabeculectomy (and its variations) and tube shunt surgery are indicated when other therapies cannot maintain the IOP at a level considered low enough to prevent further disease progression. The glaucoma may be uncontrolled for various reasons:

- Maximally tolerated medical therapy and laser surgery (trabeculoplasty, iridotomy, and/or iridoplasty/gonioplasty, when indicated) fail to adequately reduce IOP.
- Glaucomatous optic neuropathy or visual field loss is progressing despite apparent "adequate" reduction of IOP with medical therapy (with or without laser surgery).
- The patient cannot adhere to the necessary medical regimen.

Trabeculectomy

The trabeculectomy is a fistulizing procedure. It creates a new pathway (fistula) that allows aqueous humor to flow out of the anterior chamber through a surgical corneoscleral opening and into the subconjunctival and the sub-Tenon space. In the contemporary trabeculectomy, the fistula is created under a partial-thickness flap. The procedure is traditionally referred to as *filtering surgery* even though there is no filtering action.

Indications

Incisional surgery is indicated when maximally tolerated core medical therapy and laser treatment fail or are insufficient to prevent progressive damage. However, because of the potential complications of incisional glaucoma surgery (discussed later), it is not reasonable to perform trabeculectomy in an eye with ocular hypertension and a low risk of developing functional loss. In less clear-cut situations—for example, when one eye has sustained significant glaucomatous damage and the IOP is high in the fellow eye despite maximally tolerated medical therapy—some surgeons would recommend surgery prior to unequivocal detection of damage.

Failure of medical therapy may be the result of poor patient adherence, in itself a relative indication for surgery. Some patients may use their medications only shortly before an office visit. Thus, there may be progression despite apparently acceptable IOP. It is difficult to elicit an accurate history in this situation. When the ophthalmologist suspects poor patient adherence, it may be appropriate to advance to surgery sooner, because further changes in medical therapy are unlikely to improve IOP control.

The main indications for surgery are progression of visual field damage and uncontrolled IOP. Multiple visual field examinations may be required in order to confirm progression. In many cases, the decision to proceed with surgery is made even in the absence of documented progression and is based on a clinical judgment that the IOP is too high for the stage of the disease. Thus, an IOP of 25 mm Hg is not an indication for surgery in an eye with ocular hypertension, but this IOP level might be an indication for IOP-lowering surgery in the setting of advanced glaucomatous optic neuropathy. It is not always necessary to perform LTP before proceeding to trabeculectomy.

Stiles MC. Update on glaucoma surgery. *Focal Points: Clinical Modules for Ophthalmologists.* San Francisco: American Academy of Ophthalmology; 2012, module 6.

Contraindications

Relative contraindications for trabeculectomy can be ocular or systemic. A blind eye is not considered for incisional surgery. Cyclodestruction is a better alternative for lowering IOP in such eyes. The risk of sympathetic ophthalmia should always be kept in mind when any procedure on a blind eye or an eye with poor visual potential is considered. Conditions that predispose to trabeculectomy failure, such as active anterior segment neovascularization (rubeosis iridis) or active anterior uveitis, are relative contraindications. The underlying problem should be addressed first, if possible, or a surgical alternative such as implantation of a tube shunt should be considered. It may be extremely difficult to perform a successful trabeculectomy in an eye that has sustained extensive conjunctival injury (eg, after retinal detachment surgery or chemical trauma) or that has an extremely thin sclera from prior surgery or necrotizing scleritis. In such cases the likelihood of success is also reduced because of an increased risk of scarring.

The success rate of trabeculectomy is lower in younger patients or in aphakic or pseudophakic patients who have had cataract extraction through a scleral tunnel incision. However, with the advent of clear cornea phacoemulsification for cataract extraction and the use of antifibrotic agents during trabeculectomy, surgery has resulted in significant improvements in IOP in pseudophakic patients. A lower success rate is also found in patients with certain types of secondary glaucoma and in those who previously had unsuccessful filtering procedures. In addition, black patients have a higher failure rate with filtering surgery.

Fontana H, Nouri-Mahdavi K, Caprioli J. Trabeculectomy with mitomycin C in pseudophakic patients with open-angle glaucoma: outcomes and risk factors for failure. *Am J Ophthalmol.* 2006;141(4):652–659.

Shingleton BJ, Alfano C, O'Donoghue MW, Rivera J. Efficacy of glaucoma filtration surgery in pseudophakic patients with or without conjunctival scarring. *J Cataract Refract Surg.* 2004;30(12):2504–2509.

Preoperative evaluation

When considering a surgical procedure, the ophthalmologist must take into account factors such as the patient's general health, presumed life expectancy, and status of the fellow eye. The patient must be medically stable enough to endure an invasive ocular procedure under local anesthesia. The preoperative evaluation should determine and document factors that may affect surgical planning, as well as those that determine the structural and functional status of the eye.

Control of preoperative inflammation with corticosteroids helps reduce postoperative anterior uveitis and scarring of the filtering bleb. Discontinuation of anticholinesterase agents (in the rare instances when they are used), with temporary use of alternative medications, at least 3–6 weeks before surgery helps reduce bleeding and iridocyclitis. If there is an allergic dermatoconjunctivitis with severe inflammation, stopping all offending topical drops and controlling IOP with oral CAIs temporarily can be helpful. Blepharitis should be controlled preoperatively.

Before surgery, the IOP should be reduced as closely as possible to normal levels in order to minimize the risk of expulsive choroidal hemorrhage. If possible, discontinue antiplatelet and anticoagulant medications, in consultation with the patient's primary care physician. Systemic hypertension should be controlled.

Patients should be informed of the purpose of and expectations for surgery: to arrest or delay progressive vision loss caused by their glaucoma. They should understand that glaucoma surgery alone rarely improves vision and that glaucoma medications may still need to be used postoperatively; that surgery may fail completely; that they could lose vision as a result of surgery; and that glaucoma may progress despite successful surgery.

It is important to note that a patient with very advanced visual field loss or field loss that is impinging on fixation is at risk, in rare instances, of loss of central acuity after a surgical procedure. The most common cause of vision loss after trabeculectomy is cataract development. Hypotony maculopathy and cystoid macular edema may also cause vision loss. Loss of central vision in the absence of other explanations ("wipeout") may occur, but only in rare instances. Advanced age, preoperative visual field with macular splitting, and early postoperative hypotony are risk factors for wipeout. Early, undetected, postoperative elevation of IOP may also be associated with wipeout. Bleb infections and endophthalmitis may occur long after filtering surgery and may also cause vision loss.

Francis BA, Hong B, Winarko J, Kawji S, Dustin L, Chopra V. Vision loss and recovery after trabeculectomy: risk and associated risk factors. *Arch Ophthalmol.* 2011;129(8):1011–1017.

Law SK, Nguyen AM, Coleman AL, Caprioli J. Severe loss of central vision in patients with advanced glaucoma undergoing trabeculectomy. *Arch Ophthalmol.* 2007;125(8):1044–1050.

Trabeculectomy technique

Knowledge of the internal and external anatomy of the limbal area is essential for successful surgery. Trabeculectomy is a guarded partial-thickness filtering procedure in which a block of peripheral corneoscleral tissue is removed beneath a scleral flap (Video 8-1). The scleral flap provides resistance and limits the outflow of aqueous, thereby reducing the complications associated with early hypotony, such as flat anterior chamber, cataract, serous choroidal effusion and hemorrhagic choroidal detachment, hypotony maculopathy, and optic nerve edema. The use of antifibrotic agents (discussed in more detail later), such as mitomycin C (MMC) and 5-fluorouracil (5-FU), along with releasable sutures or laser suture lysis, prolongs the duration of successful IOP control.

 VIDEO 8-1 Fornix-based trabeculectomy with running closure.
Courtesy of James A. Savage, MD.
Access all Section 10 videos at www.aao.org/bcscvideo_section10.

In contrast to cataract surgery, the success of trabeculectomy is largely dependent on timely postoperative interventions that modulate wound healing of the filter site to achieve appropriate flow through the artificial aqueous outflow pathway. The goal of this procedure is complete healing of the conjunctival incision, without scarring of the scleral flap to the scleral bed and without excessive subconjunctival scarring.

A trabeculectomy can be broken down into several basic steps:

- *Exposure:* A corneal or limbal traction suture can rotate the globe downward, providing excellent exposure of the superior sulcus and limbus, which can be very helpful for a limbus-based conjunctival flap (Fig 8-4). A superior rectus bridle suture has the same effect but is more likely to cause postoperative ptosis and subconjunctival hemorrhage. The speculum should be adjusted to keep pressure off the globe.

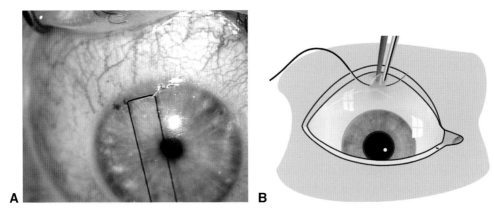

A   **B**

Figure 8-4 Exposure for trabeculectomy: a corneal traction suture **(A)** or superior rectus bridle suture **(B)** is inserted. *(Part A courtesy of Keith Barton, MD; part B courtesy of Alan Lacey. Both parts reproduced with permission of Moorfields Eye Hospital.)*

- *Conjunctival incision:* Traditionally, the trabeculectomy has been positioned at the 12 o'clock meridian or in either superior quadrant, depending on surgeon preference. There is evidence that with the use of antifibrotic agents, the trabeculectomy bleb should be positioned at the 12 o'clock meridian to reduce the risk of bleb exposure and dysesthesia. A fornix- or limbus-based conjunctival flap can be used (Figs 8-5, 8-6). Each technique has advantages and disadvantages. The fornix-based flap is easier to fashion but requires very careful suturing to achieve a watertight closure at the end of the procedure. The advantage of a fornix-based conjunctival flap is the development of a subconjunctival scar anterior to the scleral flap, which encourages posterior aqueous flow and formation of a more posterior bleb. The limbus-based conjunctival flap is technically more challenging, but it permits a secure closure well away from the limbus. The incision should be positioned 8–10 mm posterior to the limbus, and care should be taken to avoid the tendon of the superior rectus muscle. The advantage of a limbus-based flap is that it has a reduced risk of postoperative incision leakage; a potential disadvantage is the possible creation of a subconjunctival scar posterior to the scleral flap, impeding posterior flow of aqueous and encouraging more localized bleb formation closer to the limbus.

  The clinical situation will influence the placement of the conjunctival incision. For instance, in deep-set eyes with tight orbits, it may be anatomically difficult to create a limbus-based conjunctival flap. For a patient traveling long distances for postoperative care, the surgeon may elect to create a limbus-based conjunctival flap, reducing the risk of postoperative incision leakage and the number of postoperative visits that would be required to treat it.

- *Scleral flap:* The scleral flap and its relationship to the underlying sclerostomy (discussed later) provide resistance to outflow; the specific size and shape of the flap are not critical. Flap design varies according to surgeon preference, but a common technique involves creating a 3- to 4-mm triangular, trapezoidal, or rectangular flap (Fig 8-7). If a fornix-based conjunctival flap is used, it is best to avoid

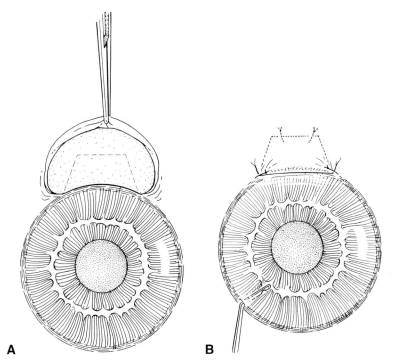

Figure 8-5 Fornix-based conjunctival flap. **A,** The drawing shows the initial incision through conjunctiva at the limbus and the insertion of the Tenon capsule. The arc length of the initial incision is approximately 6–7 mm. The tissue adjacent to the incision is undermined with blunt scissors before the scleral flap is prepared. **B,** The incision is closed either at both ends with interrupted sutures or purse-string sutures or with a running mattress suture. *(Modified with permission from Weinreb RN, Mills RP, eds.* Glaucoma Surgery: Principles and Techniques. *2nd ed. Ophthalmology Monograph 4. San Francisco: American Academy of Ophthalmology; 1998:43.)*

dissecting the flap anteriorly into clear cornea, because anterior flap dissection facilitates early wound leakage.

- *Paracentesis* (Fig 8-8): To enable the surgeon to control the anterior chamber, a paracentesis should be performed next. This allows instillation of balanced salt ophthalmic solution or viscoelastic and intraoperative testing of the patency of the filtration site. Balanced salt ophthalmic solution is instilled through the paracentesis incision, and suture tension is titrated until flow is minimal. If a postoperative flat chamber occurs, the paracentesis is already in place and can be used to re-form the chamber. Using the existing paracentesis is much safer than trying to create a paracentesis in an eye with a flat chamber.

- *Keratectomy:* In a strict sense, the term *trabeculectomy* is inaccurate because peripheral posterior cornea rather than trabecular meshwork is removed in this procedure. There is no advantage to extending the block posteriorly into sclera, and the risk of bleeding from the iris root and ciliary body is greater. The keratectomy is commonly performed with the use of a punch, although a block may also be cut with a fine blade (Fig 8-9). Aqueous drainage is generally not restricted by the size of the opening. A very small hole can drain more aqueous than is required to control

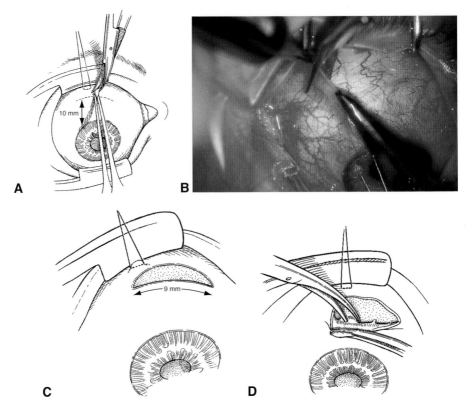

Figure 8-6 Limbus-based conjunctival flap. **A,** The drawing shows the initial incision through conjunctiva and Tenon capsule. **B,** Clinical photograph corresponding to part A shows the initial incision for creation of a limbus-based conjunctival flap. **C,** Completion of conjunctiva–Tenon incision 8–10 mm posterior to the limbus. **D,** Anterior dissection of conjunctiva–Tenon flap with excision of Tenon episcleral fibrous adhesions. *(Parts A, C, and D modified with permission from Weinreb RN, Mills RP, eds.* Glaucoma Surgery: Principles and Techniques. *2nd ed. Ophthalmology Monograph 4. San Francisco: American Academy of Ophthalmology; 1998:29–31. Part B courtesy of Robert D. Fechtner, MD.)*

IOP. However, the keratectomy must be large enough to avoid occlusion by iris, but small enough so that it is overlapped on all sides by scleral flap. Insertion of a small titanium shunt under the flap, in lieu of a keratectomy can standardize the size of the hole for drainage and avoid a freehand keratectomy. More overlap, a thicker flap, and tighter sutures are generally associated with less flow; the converse is also true.

- *Iridectomy:* An iridectomy is performed to reduce the risk of iris occluding the sclerostomy, especially in phakic and narrow-angle eyes, and to prevent pupillary block (see Fig 8-9D). An iridectomy may not always be necessary in pseudophakic eyes with deep anterior chambers. Care should be taken to avoid amputation of the ciliary processes or disruption of the zonular fibers or hyaloid face. If a titanium shunt is inserted under the flap, an iridectomy is not necessary.

- *Closure of scleral flap:* The flap is reapproximated to its bed with 10-0 or 9-0 nylon (Fig 8-10). With the advent of laser suture lysis and releasable sutures (discussed later under "Flap management"), many surgeons close the flap more tightly, thereby

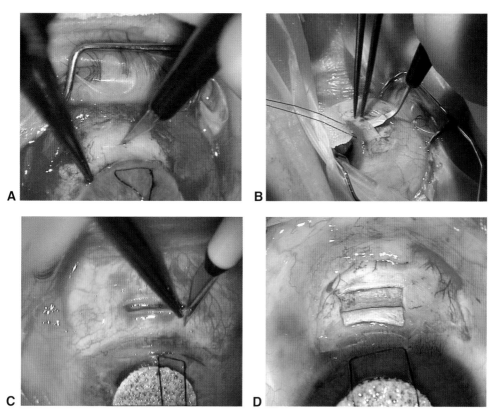

Figure 8-7 Clinical photographs showing creation of the scleral flap. Preparation of a scleral flap 4 mm wide and 2–2.5 mm from front to back at 50%–75% scleral depth. **A,** The posterior margin is dissected with a fine blade. **B,** A crescent knife is used to dissect a partial-thickness scleral tunnel. **C,** The sides of the tunnel are opened to create a flap. **D,** The final appearance. *(Courtesy of Keith Barton, MD. Reproduced with permission of Moorfields Eye Hospital.)*

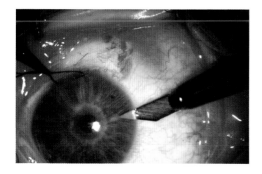

Figure 8-8 A paracentesis is created through clear cornea, radial to the limbus. *(Courtesy of Keith Barton, MD. Reproduced with permission of Moorfields Eye Hospital.)*

minimizing postoperative shallowing of the anterior chamber. After a few days or weeks, these techniques can release tension on the flap and promote flow. It is important to test the integrity of the scleral flap before closing the conjunctiva. When MMC is used, tension and number of sutures should be adjusted until optimal spontaneous flow can be seen. To ensure that suture adjustment will further

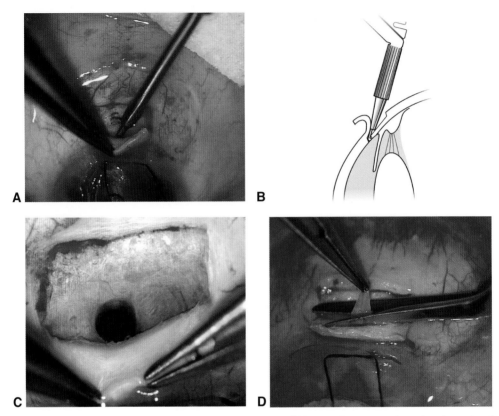

Figure 8-9 The surgeon can create a keratectomy by **(A)** inserting a punch under the scleral flap; **(B)** snaring the posterior lip of the anterior chamber entry site; and **(C)** removing a punch (0.75–1 mm) of peripheral posterior cornea. A peripheral iridectomy is then made (shown here in an albino eye) with the use of iridectomy scissors **(D)**. *(Clinical photographs courtesy of Keith Barton, MD; illustration based on original drawing by Alan Lacey. All parts reproduced with permission of Moorfields Eye Hospital.)*

increase outflow, the surgeon can test the flow. It should be possible to induce additional flow with gentle depression of the posterior scleral lip.

- *Closure of conjunctiva:* Many techniques have been developed for conjunctival closure (Fig 8-11). It is imperative that the closure be watertight at the completion of the procedure. For a fornix-based flap, conjunctiva is secured at the limbus. Several techniques are used for this closure, including episcleral-anchored interrupted sutures at each end of the incision; a running mattress suture; and purse-string closures at each end of the incision, with or without mattress sutures in between. For a limbus-based flap, conjunctiva and Tenon capsule are closed separately or in a single layer with a running suture of 9-0 nylon or polyglactin 910 on a vascular needle, which minimizes wound leak in procedures where MMC has been applied.

Jones E, Clarke J, Khaw PT. Recent advances in trabeculectomy technique. *Curr Opin Ophthalmol.* 2005;16(2):107–113.

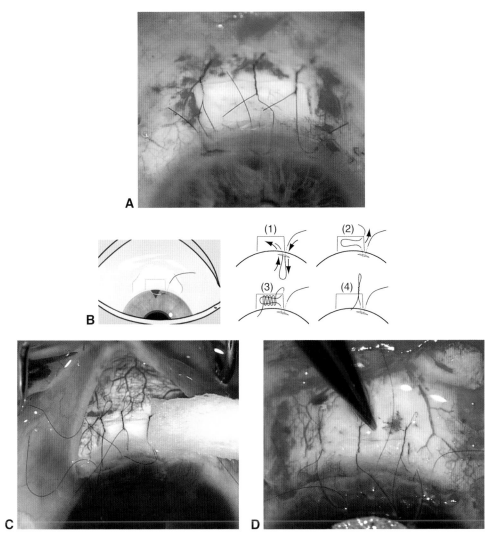

Figure 8-10 In a mitomycin C (MMC) trabeculectomy, the scleral flap is closed relatively tightly so that spontaneous drainage is minimal. Closure may be performed with the use of releasable sutures **(A, B)** that can be removed later at the slit lamp in order to increase flow, or with interrupted sutures that may be cut by laser postoperatively. **B** shows the order in which each movement is made to place one type of releasable suture. The surgeon should check the flow at the end of scleral closure using a sponge **(C)** or fluorescein **(D)**. *(Clinical photographs courtesy of Keith Barton, MD; drawing courtesy of Alan Lacey. All parts reproduced with permission of Moorfields Eye Hospital.)*

Antifibrotic agents

The application of antifibrotic agents such as 5-FU and MMC results in lower IOP following trabeculectomy. However, the rate of serious postoperative complications may be higher, and these agents must not be used indiscriminately. Because their use is associated with an increased risk of hypotony maculopathy, antifibrotic agents should be used with caution in primary trabeculectomies on young patients with myopia.

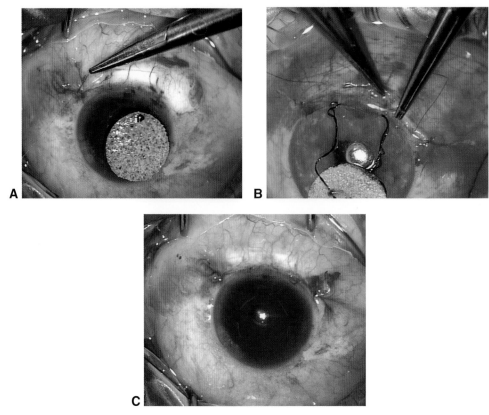

Figure 8-11 Clinical photographs showing conjunctival closure. Careful conjunctival closure is essential to prevent aqueous leakage, especially when a fornix-based conjunctival flap is used. Closing each extremity of the incision tightly with a purse-string suture **(A)** stretches the limbal edge of the conjunctiva, facilitating tight closure at the limbus. One or more conjunctival mattress sutures **(B)** prevent conjunctival recession. **C** shows an inflated bleb. *(Courtesy of Keith Barton, MD. Reproduced with permission of Moorfields Eye Hospital.)*

The pyrimidine analogue 5-FU reversibly inhibits fibroblast proliferation and has proven useful in reducing scarring after filtering surgery. The agent undergoes intracellular conversion to the active deoxynucleotide 5-fluoro-2′-deoxyuridine 5′-monophosphate (FdUMP), which interferes with DNA synthesis through its action on thymidylate synthetase.

Although 5-FU was originally advocated for use in high-risk groups such as patients with aphakic or pseudophakic eyes, neovascular glaucoma, or a history of failed operations, many surgeons now use 5-FU on a routine basis. This agent can be used intraoperatively (50 mg/mL on a surgical sponge) in a fashion similar to that described next for MMC. Regimens for postoperative administration vary according to the observed healing response. Individual doses of 5–10 mg in 0.1–0.5 mL can be injected. The total dose can be titrated to the observed healing response and corneal toxicity. Complications such as corneal epithelial defects commonly occur and require discontinuation of 5-FU injections. The site of the 5-FU injection can be varied: either 180° away from the trabeculectomy site or in the upper fornix adjacent to the bleb. As this agent is highly alkaline, the surgeon should avoid injecting 5-FU close to the scleral flap to reduce the risk of intra-ocular exposure.

Derived from *Streptomyces caespitosus*, MMC is a naturally occurring compound with antibiotic and antineoplastic activities. It acts as an alkylating agent after enzyme activation, resulting in DNA crosslinking. MMC is a potent antifibrotic agent that is most commonly administered intraoperatively in the following manner: a surgical sponge soaked in MMC is placed within the subconjunctival space so that it is in contact with sclera at the planned trabeculectomy site. Concentrations in current usage are typically 0.1–0.5 mg/mL with a duration of application from 0.5 to 5 minutes. Most surgeons use the higher concentrations for shorter durations and vice versa. Few data are available to compare regimens, and most surgeons increase concentration or duration based on risk factors for trabeculectomy failure. The technique of MMC application has evolved to cover a larger area with increased posterior exposure in an attempt to develop a more diffuse, low-lying bleb (Fig 8-12) instead of a localized, elevated bleb (Fig 8-13), which is inherently at greater risk of infection. Alternatively, instead of using a pledget, many surgeons inject MMC subconjunctivally before surgery to achieve a diffuse application. Doses ranging from 5 to 30 μg have been used. Because MMC is toxic and highly mutagenic, intracameral exposure must be avoided.

Flap management

Techniques allowing tighter initial closure of the scleral flap help prevent early postoperative hypotony. Two of these techniques are the use of releasable flap sutures (Video 8-2) and the placement of additional sutures that can be cut postoperatively to facilitate outflow following trabeculectomy. In laser suture lysis (LSL), the conjunctiva is compressed

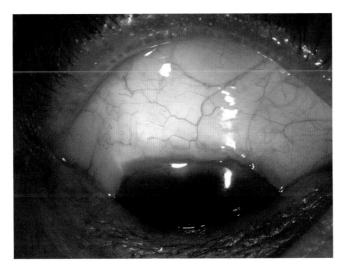

Figure 8-12 Clinical photograph showing diffuse conjunctival bleb. It is difficult to recognize that there is a bleb, but clues are the irregular conjunctival border at the limbus and scarring at the 10- and 2-o'clock positions, where sutures were placed during surgery. Also, with careful slit-lamp examination, one will notice that the bleb is elevated off the sclera. *(Courtesy of JoAnn Giaconi, MD.)*

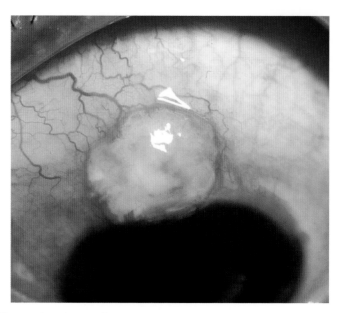

Figure 8-13 Clinical photograph of a localized conjunctival bleb. *(Courtesy of Jody Piltz-Seymour, MD.)*

with either a Zeiss goniolens or a lens designed for suture lysis (such as a Hoskins, Ritch, Mandelkorn, or Blumenthal lens), and the argon green laser (set at 240–600 mW at a duration of 0.02–0.1 second with a spot size of 50–100 μm) or red laser can usually lyse the selected black 10-0 nylon suture with one application. It is important to avoid creating a full-thickness conjunctival burn. Shorter duration of laser energy and avoidance of pigment or blood are helpful for preventing such a burn. Most surgeons wait at least 48 hours before performing LSL. Filtration is best enhanced if lysis or suture release is completed within 2–4 weeks of the surgery or before the occurrence of flap fibrosis. This period may be lengthened to several months when antifibrotic agents have been used.

 VIDEO 8-2 Placement of a releasable suture for flap closure.
Courtesy of Marlene Moster, MD.

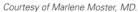

Postoperative considerations in trabeculectomy

The success of glaucoma surgery depends on careful postoperative management. In general, glaucoma medications are stopped for the surgical eye. If oral CAIs are discontinued, an adjustment in medication may be necessary for the fellow eye. Topical corticosteroids are typically administered intensively (at least 4 times daily) initially and tapered as the clinical course dictates. Topical antibiotics or cycloplegic agents may also be used. Topical corticosteroids should be tapered according to the degree of conjunctival hyperemia, which may continue for 2 months or more, rather than in response to the visible anterior chamber reaction, which usually resolves more quickly. Long-term use of prophylactic antibiotics is generally not recommended. Trabeculectomies require intensive early postoperative care, and frequent office visits are necessary in the first postoperative month. During this period, if the IOP is above target, it is common for the clinician to do the following: prescribe digital ocular pressure (for 2 seconds a pulse in multiples of 3–10 twice daily); administer 5-FU injections; and/or lyse permanent sutures or remove releasable sutures. An advantage of frequent visits in the early postoperative period is that if hypotony or a flat chamber occurs, it will not go undiagnosed for a prolonged period.

Complications of trabeculectomy

Early and late complications of filtering surgery are listed in Table 8-1. Early complications include wound leaks at incision sites, hypotony, shallow or flat anterior chamber, and serous or hemorrhagic choroidal effusions. Late complications include blebitis, bleb-related endophthalmitis, bleb leakage, hypotony and associated maculopathy or choroidal hemorrhage, bleb failure, overhanging blebs, painful blebs, ptosis, and eyelid retraction. The filtering bleb can leak, produce dellen, or expand so as to interfere with eyelid function or extend onto the cornea and interfere with vision or cause irritation. Blebs may also encapsulate or fibrose, causing elevated IOP. Filtering blebs are dynamic; they evolve over time and must be monitored. All patients must be informed of the warning signs of bleb-related infections and instructed to seek ophthalmic care immediately should they develop a red eye or other signs of infection.

Late-onset bleb-related endophthalmitis is a potentially devastating complication of filtering surgery. In adults, the incidence of postoperative endophthalmitis associated with glaucoma surgery with or without antifibrotic drugs has been reported to range from 1.3% per patient-year for superior blebs to 7.8% per patient-year for inferior blebs. Risk factors for bleb-related endophthalmitis include blepharitis or conjunctivitis, ocular trauma, nasolacrimal duct obstruction, contact lens use, chronic bleb leak, male sex, and young age. Trabeculectomy performed at the inferior limbus is associated with an unacceptably high risk of bleb-related endophthalmitis. Use of adjunctive antifibrotic drugs such as 5-FU or MMC has been associated with an increased risk of bleb-related endophthalmitis, perhaps because these blebs are often thin-walled and avascular. Patients may present with blebitis or with blebitis and endophthalmitis (Fig 8-14).

Table 8-1 Complications of Trabeculectomy

Early Complications	Late Complications
Choroidal effusion	Cataract
Cystoid macular edema	Bleb migration
Dellen formation	Blebitis
Formation or acceleration of cataract	Endophthalmitis/bleb infection
Hyphema	Eyelid retraction
Hypotony	Hypotony
Hypotony maculopathy	Leakage or failure of the filtering bleb
Infection	Ptosis
Loss of vision	Symptomatic bleb (dysesthetic bleb)
Malignant glaucoma (aqueous misdirection)	
Persistent uveitis	
Shallow or flat anterior chamber	
Suprachoroidal hemorrhage	
Transient IOP elevation	
Wound leak	

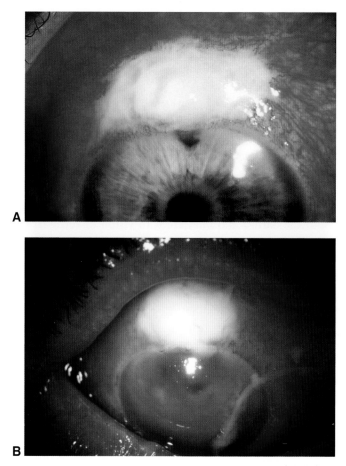

Figure 8-14 Bleb-related infection. Patients may present with blebitis, which is characterized by mucopurulent infiltrate within the bleb, localized conjunctival hyperemia, and minimal intraocular inflammation **(A)**. Bleb-related endophthalmitis **(B)** is characterized by diffuse bulbar conjunctival hyperemia, purulent material within the bleb, and anterior chamber cellular reaction; it is also sometimes characterized by hypopyon formation and marked vitritis. *(Part A courtesy of Richard K. Parrish, MD; part B courtesy of Keith Barton, MD. Part B is reproduced with permission of Moorfields Eye Hospital.)*

Hypotony after filtering surgery is usually due to overfiltration through the scleral flap and can be associated with bleb leaks. Aqueous leakage from a filtering bleb may occur as an early or late complication of surgery. Early-onset bleb leaks are usually related to ineffective wound closure or a conjunctival buttonhole. Late-onset leaks occur more frequently after full-thickness procedures such as posterior lip sclerectomy or after use of antifibrotic drugs. Untreated bleb leaks may lead to vision-threatening complications, including shallowing of the anterior chamber, PAS formation, cataract, corneal decompensation, choroidal effusion, suprachoroidal hemorrhage, endophthalmitis, and hypotony maculopathy. Clinical manifestations of hypotony maculopathy include decreased vision, hypotony, optic nerve and retinal edema, and radial folds of the macula.

Choroidal effusions are more likely to occur in elderly patients because of increased scleral rigidity, which occurs with age and does not allow sclera to buckle under low pressure. Eyes with thin, pliable sclera tend to develop hypotony maculopathy. Choroidal effusions may be treated medically with cycloplegics, with injection of a viscoelastic substance into the anterior chamber, or by choroidal drainage. Suprachoroidal fluid can be drained through one or more posterior full-thickness sclerotomies overlying the area of effusion, as the anterior chamber is deepened through a paracentesis.

Numerous techniques have been described for managing bleb leaks, including the use of an oversize contact lens, aqueous suppressants, suture, tissue glue, autologous blood injection, and oral antibiotics from the tetracycline family. Excision of the bleb, in combination with a conjunctival graft or conjunctival advancement with or without a scleral graft, is also possible. The surgeon may also advance a conjunctival flap over the existing bleb. If there is undue tension during closure, conjunctival relaxing incisions and a pedicle conjunctival flap can be created to help closure.

The bleb may fail following filtering surgery. In eyes with failing blebs, reduced bleb height, increased bleb-wall thickness, vascularization of the bleb, loss of conjunctival microcysts, and increased IOP may be seen. Risk factors for bleb failure include anterior segment neovascularization, black race, aphakia, prior failed filtering procedures, uveitis, prior cataract surgery, prior vitreoretinal surgery, and young age. Initial management of failing blebs often includes digital pressure. In eyes that do not respond to this initial therapy, transconjunctival needle revision may restore aqueous flow.

The use of contact lenses with a filtering bleb presents special problems. Contact lenses may be difficult to fit in the presence of a filtering bleb, or the lens may ride against the bleb, causing discomfort and increasing the risk of infection. Several options can be considered for the patient who has myopia, requires a trabeculectomy, and prefers not to or cannot wear spectacles. Clear lens extraction (either before, after, or combined with trabeculectomy) is controversial. In some circumstances, hard or soft contact lens use under close supervision may be considered after trabeculectomy. Contact lens use is more often feasible in patients after tube shunt implantation than after trabeculectomy. When an initial filtering procedure is not adequate to control the glaucoma and resumption of medical therapy is not successful, revision of original surgery, a second filtering surgery at a new site, tube shunt implantation, or possibly cyclodestructive procedures may be indicated.

DeBry PW, Perkins TW, Heatley G, Kaufman P, Brumback LC. Incidence of late-onset bleb-related complications following trabeculectomy with mitomycin. *Arch Ophthalmol.* 2002; 120(3):297–300.

Haynes WL, Alward WL. Control of intraocular pressure after trabeculectomy. *Surv Ophthalmol.* 1999;43(4):345–355.

Tannenbaum DP, Hoffman D, Greaney MJ, Caprioli J. Outcomes of bleb excision and conjunctival advancement for leaking or hypotonous eyes after glaucoma filtering surgery. *Br J Ophthalmol.* 2004;88(1):99–103.

Combined Cataract and Trabeculectomy

Both cataract and glaucoma are conditions that are more prevalent with age. It is not surprising that many patients with glaucoma eventually develop cataracts either naturally or as a result of glaucoma therapy. It should also be noted that cataract surgery alone may lower IOP in eyes with open angles and may lower it even more in eyes with phacomorphic narrow angles. However, cataract surgery as a treatment of open-angle glaucoma is a topic of debate.

A combined procedure (cataract extraction plus trabeculectomy) may prevent a post-operative rise in IOP. Combined procedures are generally less effective than trabeculectomy alone in controlling IOP over time because the inflammation induced by cataract surgery increases the risk of bleb failure. For patients in whom glaucoma is the greatest immediate threat to vision, trabeculectomy alone is usually performed first.

Several clinical challenges are common in patients with coexisting cataract and glaucoma. Medical therapy for glaucoma may create chronic miosis, and the surgeon must deal with a small pupil. The anterior chamber can be very shallow in eyes with angle closure, making cataract surgery technically difficult. In patients with pseudoexfoliation syndrome, zonular support of the lens is often fragile, and vitreous loss is therefore more common in such complicated eyes. As with all surgery, the risks, benefits, and alternatives should be discussed with the patient.

Indications

Cataract surgery may be combined with trabeculectomy in the following situations:

- cataract requiring extraction in a glaucoma patient who has advanced cupping and visual field loss to minimize postoperative pressure spike
- cataract requiring extraction in a glaucoma patient who requires medications to control IOP but who tolerates medical therapy poorly or has inadequately controlled IOP
- cataract requiring extraction in a glaucoma patient who requires multiple medications to control IOP

As stated earlier, combined procedures are generally less effective than trabeculectomy alone in controlling IOP. Thus, in uncontrolled glaucoma, combined surgery is usually performed only in specific circumstances, such as primary angle-closure glaucoma uncontrolled with medications or after laser iridotomy when cataract surgery alone is unlikely to provide successful IOP control. Many surgeons perform trabeculectomy with cataract surgery when the IOP is stable but the patient is using 2 or 3 IOP-lowering medications. The goal in these cases is to avoid perioperative problems with elevated IOP and to achieve a long-term reduction in the number of medications required. However, many surgeons would perform cataract surgery alone in a patient who has controlled IOP using 1 medication, with mild to moderate cupping and little visual field loss.

Relative contraindications

Combined cataract and filtering surgery should be avoided in the following situations, in which glaucoma surgery alone is preferred:

- glaucoma that requires a very low target IOP
- advanced glaucoma with uncontrolled IOP and immediate need for successful reduction of IOP

Technique

Several surgical approaches to coexisting cataract and glaucoma are currently used. Although little evidence exists to compare the long-term outcomes of patients treated with these different approaches, it is reasonable for the surgeon to use the cataract procedure that he or she performs best, because the primary indication for surgery is the presence of cataract.

Trabeculectomy may be combined with phacoemulsification, which is performed through the superior trabeculectomy incision or through a temporal clear corneal incision. Also, cataract extraction may be combined with implantation of a tube shunt. In addition, there are several procedures that combine cataract surgery with surgery on the Schlemm canal, such as canaloplasty (see the section Nonpenetrating Glaucoma Surgery), implantation of a trabecular microbypass stent (eg, iStent, Glaukos Corp, Laguna Hills, CA), and ab interno trabeculotomy with an electroablation device (eg, Trabectome, NeoMedix Inc, Tustin, CA). Electroablation of the trabecular meshwork is performed through a temporal corneal incision, a technique similar to that used in goniotomy, to lower IOP in open-angle glaucoma.

For the patient whose IOP is controlled medically, clear corneal cataract surgery alone may be the appropriate choice. As no violation of conjunctiva or sclera occurs with this procedure, standard trabeculectomy can be performed later when dictated by independent indications.

Augustinus CJ, Zeyen T. The effect of phacoemulsification and combined phaco/glaucoma procedures on the intraocular pressure in open-angle glaucoma. A review of the literature. *Bull Soc Belge Ophthalmol.* 2012;320:51–66.

Jin GJ, Crandall AS, Jones JJ. Phacotrabeculectomy: assessment of outcomes and surgical improvements. *J Cataract Refract Surg.* 2007;33(7):1201–1208.

Cataract Extraction

Cataract extraction has been shown, on average, to lower IOP in eyes with ocular hypertension and various types of glaucoma. This ocular hypotensive effect does decrease over time. In eyes with open angles, IOP reduction resulting from cataract extraction can be equivalent to the pressure-lowering effect achieved with one hypotensive eyedrop, and the greatest reductions are seen in eyes with higher pressures. When pupillary block is associated with a visually significant cataract, lens extraction might be considered as a primary procedure to relieve pupillary block. However, laser iridotomy can be considered as a first step to stop acute pupillary block, so that cataract surgery may be performed more safely at a later time. Cataract extraction combined with goniosynechialysis may be effective in patients with chronic angle-closure following acute PAC and in patients with PAC unresponsive to laser iridotomy.

Harasymowycz PJ, Papamatheakis DG, Ahmed I, et al. Phacoemulsification and goniosynechialysis in the management of unresponsive primary angle closure. *J Glaucoma.* 2005; 14(3):186–189.

Mansberger SL, Gordon MO, Jampel H, et al. Reduction in intraocular pressure after cataract extraction: the Ocular Hypertension Treatment Study. *Ophthalmology.* 2012;119(9):1826–1831.

Tube Shunt Implantation

There are many different types of devices that aid angle filtration by shunting aqueous to a site away from the limbus, such as the equatorial subconjunctival space. Tube shunt implantation generally involves placing a tube in the anterior chamber, in the ciliary sulcus, or through the pars plana into the vitreous cavity. The tube is connected to an extraocular plate, which is attached to the sclera in the equatorial region of the globe, between the extraocular muscles, and in some cases tucked under the muscles; some devices employ 2 plates. Aqueous flows out through the tube and into the subconjunctival space in the region of the extraocular plate.

Tube shunts can be broadly categorized as *nonvalved devices,* which have no flow restrictor, or *valved devices,* which have a flow restrictor (Table 8-2). The most frequently used nonvalved devices are the Molteno (Molteno Ophthalmic Ltd, Dunedin, New Zealand) and Baerveldt (Abbott Medical Optics, Santa Ana, CA) designs. The most widely used valved device is the Ahmed design (New World Medical, Inc, Rancho Cucamonga, CA). Two multicenter randomized controlled trials comparing the Ahmed glaucoma valve (AGV) and the Baerveldt glaucoma implant (BGI) found that the average IOP after 3–5 years was slightly higher in patients who received the AGV; however, there were fewer vision-threatening complications associated with use of the AGV than with the BGI. The surface area of the plate of each tube shunt varies and can influence IOP control and complications postoperatively.

In eyes with an existing encircling band placed for retinal detachment, a Schocket procedure can be performed. In this procedure, a silicone tube is passed from the anterior chamber and threaded into the capsule surrounding a previously placed scleral buckle (Video 8-3).

 VIDEO 8-3   Schocket procedure.
Courtesy of Herbert P. Fechter III, MD.

Budenz DL, Barton K, Gedde SJ, et al. Five-year treatment outcomes in the Ahmed Baerveldt comparison study. *Ophthalmology.* 2015;122(2):308–316.

Indications

The devices mentioned and similar types of implants have generally been reserved for difficult glaucoma cases in which trabeculectomy has failed or is likely to fail. However, tube shunt implantation can be used as a primary procedure. The 5-year follow-up

Table 8-2 Tube Shunts

	Molteno			Baerveldt		Ahmed		Eagle Vision
	Single Plate	Double Plate	M3	Single Plate		Single Plate	Double Plate	Single Plate
Surface area, mm²	133	265	175 230	250	350	184	364	365
Height profile, mm	1.65	1.65	1.50	0.84	0.84	1.90	1.90	1.75
Plate material	Polypropylene			Silicone		Polypropylene or silicone		Silicone
Flow restrictor	No	No	Ridge	No	No	Yes	Yes	No
Pediatric surface area, mm²	55	–	–	–	–	96	–	–

results of the Tube Versus Trabeculectomy study showed that tube shunt surgery with a Baerveldt implant had a higher success rate compared with trabeculectomy with MMC in eyes with prior intraocular surgery. Both procedures were associated with a similar reduction in IOP and use of supplemental medications, but tube shunts required fewer additional surgical procedures. A tube shunt should be considered in the following clinical settings:

- *Failed trabeculectomy with antifibrotics:* It may be appropriate to perform a second trabeculectomy in some clinical situations. However, when the factors that precipitated the initial failure cannot be modified, or when it is not technically possible to repeat the trabeculectomy, implantation of a tube shunt may be the procedure of choice.
- *Active uveitis:* Although few randomized, prospective studies have been performed comparing trabeculectomy with antifibrotics to tube shunts in active uveitis, the success rate of trabeculectomy is disappointingly low in most cases of active inflammation. In certain types of uveitis (eg, young patients with juvenile idiopathic arthritis), the success rate of trabeculectomy is low and tube shunt implantation is often the primary surgical treatment.
- *Neovascular glaucoma:* Eyes with neovascular glaucoma are at high risk of trabeculectomy failure. In one prospective study, the 5-year success rate of trabeculectomy with 5-FU in neovascular glaucoma was 28%. When possible, panretinal photocoagulation and anti-VEGF therapy should be administered prior to glaucoma surgery in cases of neovascular glaucoma. When the IOP level is such that urgent surgery is required, or when the neovascular glaucoma does not respond to panretinal photocoagulation, a tube shunt is indicated. These medications may decrease the risk of perioperative intraocular bleeding.
- *Inadequate conjunctiva:* In patients who have undergone severe trauma or previous surgery involving conjunctiva (eg, retinal detachment surgery), the likelihood of trabeculectomy success may be reduced because these patients may have excessive conjunctival scarring. A tube shunt can be implanted, even in the presence of a scleral buckle. When a complete vitrectomy has been performed, the tube can be placed through the pars plana.
- *Aphakia:* The success rate of conventional filtering surgery in aphakic eyes is low, even when MMC is used. Many surgeons use tube shunts as a primary procedure in uncontrolled aphakic glaucoma. Special attention should be paid to any vitreous in an aphakic eye, as vitreous may occlude the tube.
- *Contact lens use:* The need for contact lens use for vision rehabilitation is an important consideration. The use of a soft contact lens over a trabeculectomy bleb is a risk factor for bleb trauma and subsequent infection. The use of a soft contact lens following tube shunt implantation is not without risk, however, as the conjunctiva overlying the tube is more prone to erosion with contact lens use.

Contraindications

Tube shunts may have a complicated postoperative course. Borderline corneal endothelial function is a relative contraindication for anterior chamber placement of a tube.

Preoperative considerations

The preoperative evaluation for tube shunt implantation is similar to that for trabeculec-tomy. During the ophthalmic examination, the clinician should note the findings of the motility examination, the status of the conjunctiva, the health of the sclera at the antici-pated sites for the tube and external plate, the location of PAS near possible tube insertion sites, and the location of vitreous in the eye. The clinician should also note a previously placed scleral buckle.

Techniques

Although tube shunts differ in design, the basic techniques for implantation are similar. The superotemporal quadrant is the preferred first quadrant for all models. Subsequent tube shunts can be placed in any quadrant, but the inferonasal quadrant tends to be used next for larger plate models, while the superonasal quadrant is used for smaller plate mod-els. Implantation in the superonasal quadrant may be associated with restricted eye move-ment due to impaired movement of the superior oblique tendon. If there is silicone oil in the eye, or if it is anticipated, an inferior quadrant is preferred. Valved devices must be primed before implantation (Video 8-4). The extraocular plate is sutured between the ver-tical and horizontal rectus muscles, posterior to the muscle insertions. The tube portion of the device is then routed in 1 of 3 ways: anteriorly to enter the anterior chamber angle parallel to the iris; into the ciliary sulcus in a pseudophakic eye with a posterior facing bevel entering 2.5 mm from the limbus; or through the pars plana, 4 mm to the limbus, for posterior implantation in eyes that have had a complete vitrectomy. Typically, the tube is covered with tissue such as sclera, pericardium, or cornea to help prevent erosion through the conjunctiva. Corneal patch grafts are particularly useful with inferiorly placed tubes because of a better cosmetic result. Dura should be avoided because of the potential risk of prion transmission.

 VIDEO 8-4 Ahmed valve implantation.
Courtesy of Simon K. Law, MD, PharmD.

For the nonvalved devices, there are a number of techniques to restrict flow in the early postoperative period, such as stenting the tube lumen or ligating the tube with a suture (Video 8-5). Manually restricting flow is not necessary with devices that contain a built-in flow restrictor, although hypotony and a flat chamber can still sometimes occur with them. Administering antifibrotic agents in doses similar to those used in trabecu-lectomy does not appear to improve the success of tube shunt surgery. For devices with 2 plates, the second plate and its interconnecting tube may be placed either over or under the superior rectus muscle; the distal plate is attached to the sclera in a manner similar to that in which the proximal plate is attached.

 VIDEO 8-5 Baerveldt tube shunt implantation.
Courtesy of JoAnn Giaconi, MD.

A confounding cause of hypotony can be leakage of aqueous around the tube at its entry site. In general, tubes should be introduced into the anterior chamber via a needle incision that is no larger than the diameter of the tube (23 gauge for most tubes). When the patient's eye has thin sclera or when the tube is introduced under a partial-thickness scleral flap, a tighter entry site (eg, 25 gauge) may be required.

Postoperative management

The IOP in the early postoperative period can be variable. With nonvalved devices in which the tube has been occluded, early IOP spikes are best managed medically. After sufficient time has passed for a capsule to form around the extraocular plate, the occluding suture is released or dissolves spontaneously for the nonvalved devices. As with trabeculectomy, topical corticosteroids, topical antibiotics, and cycloplegic agents are used. In valved devices, IOP elevation occurs around 2–8 weeks postoperatively, which probably represents encapsulation of the extraocular reservoir. Aqueous suppression can control the IOP, and this elevation usually improves within 1–6 months.

Complications

Success rates have been encouraging, but the implant procedures share many of the complications associated with conventional filtering surgery. In addition, unique problems related to the tubes and plates arise. Early overfiltration in an eye with tube placement in the anterior chamber results in a flat chamber and tube–cornea touch. Tube–cornea touch can compromise the cornea; and even when no touch occurs, an area of corneal decompensation can appear near the tube. Eyes must be monitored for late complications such as tube erosion or plate migration. Ocular motility disturbances may also occur. Tube obstruction, plate migration, or tube erosion may require surgical revision. Table 8-3 lists several common complications of tube shunts, along with methods for avoiding their development or managing them.

Gedde SJ, Herndon LW, Brandt JD, Budenz DL, Feuer WJ, Schiffman JC. Surgical complications in the Tube Versus Trabeculectomy Study during the first year of follow-up. *Am J Ophthalmol.* 2007;143(1):23–31.

Gedde SJ, Schiffman JC, Feuer WJ, et al. Three-year follow-up of the Tube Versus Trabeculectomy Study. *Am J Ophthalmol.* 2009;148(5):670–684.

Gedde SJ, Schiffman JC, Feuer WJ, Herndon LW, Brandt JD, Budenz DL. Treatment outcomes in the Tube Versus Trabeculectomy Study after one year of follow-up. *Am J Ophthalmol.* 2007;143(1):9–22.

Nonpenetrating Glaucoma Surgery

Nonpenetrating glaucoma procedures (deep sclerectomy) were initially described in the early 1970s. The goal was to achieve IOP lowering while avoiding some of the complications of standard trabeculectomy. Recently, interest in nonpenetrating surgery has revived. These newer nonpenetrating procedures include deep sclerectomy with or without a collagen implant, viscocanalostomy, and canaloplasty. In both viscocanalostomy and canaloplasty, a deep sclerectomy is augmented with injection of viscoelastic into the Schlemm canal. In viscocanalostomy, a cannula is used to inject viscoelastic into a limited section of the Schlemm canal. In canaloplasty, a flexible illuminated catheter is utilized to inject viscoelastic into the full 360° of the canal and to pass a suture through it; the suture is then tied, leaving the canal stretched. In deep sclerectomy, canaloplasty (Video 8-6), and viscocanalostomy, the surgeon creates a fornix-based conjunctival incision, then creates a

Table 8-3 Complications of Tube Shunt Surgery and Options for Their Prevention and Management

Complication	Prevention/Management
Tube–cornea touch	Insert tube in anterior chamber parallel to the iris plane.
	Use a tube occlusion technique to avoid flat chambers with nonvalved shunts.
	Pars plana and ciliary sulcus insertion decrease this complication.
Flat chamber and hypotony	Valved devices can decrease overfiltration leading to these complications.
	With nonvalved devices, occlusion of tube by ligature or suture within tube can decrease early hypotony.
	Use of viscoelastic agents if flat chamber develops.
	Ensure entry site of tube is watertight around the tube (ie, choose needle size to create scleral track carefully).
	Correct overdrainage early.
	Consider drainage of suprachoroidal effusions.
	Cycloplegics and corticosteroids can help deepen a shallow, but not a flat, chamber.
	A flat chamber resulting from a complication such as suprachoroidal hemorrhage must be managed based on the clinical setting.
Tube occlusion	Bevel the tube away from uveal tissue (iris) or vitreous.
	Generous vitrectomy should be performed if needed.
	Nd:YAG laser can be used to clear an occlusion; however, surgical intervention is often required.
Plate migration or tube retraction	Secure plate tightly to sclera with nonabsorbable sutures.
	If the plate migrates, the intraocular tube may become longer or retract. Plate migration toward the limbus requires repositioning of the plate in the equatorial subconjunctival space. Plate migration away from the limbus is rarely significant enough to warrant repositioning but may require a tube-extender if the tube retracts from the anterior chamber.
Valve malfunction	Test valves for patency before insertion of the tube. Several techniques have been described to unclog a valve.
Tube or plate exposure or erosion	Repair tube or plate exposure by removing any protruding sutures that have precipitated the erosion, securing tube tightly to sclera, covering tube with reinforcing material (eg, sclera, cornea, or pericardium), and mobilizing conjunctiva.
	Patch graft must be adequately covered with conjunctiva, or further erosion may occur.
	If adequate conjunctiva is not available, conjunctival autograft or amniotic membrane may be used.
	Exposure increases the risk of endophthalmitis. In some settings, the tube should be removed if adequate coverage cannot be achieved.

superficial scleral flap and next removes deeper sclera and peripheral cornea underneath, leaving only a thin layer of sclera and Descemet membrane. This allows aqueous to percolate through the Descemet membrane into a scleral lake formed by the removal of the deep scleral flap.

 VIDEO 8-6 Canaloplasty.
Courtesy of Steven Vold, MD.

These surgeries are indicated in open-angle glaucoma. Currently, there are limited long-term data from prospective, randomized trials comparing these new procedures with trabeculectomy. In theory, nonpenetrating surgery should avoid some of the complications associated with trabeculectomy. However, the procedures are technically challenging, and most results suggest that the IOP reduction achieved with nonpenetrating procedures is less than that achieved with trabeculectomy. These procedures also cause conjunctival scarring, which may limit future surgical options. Proponents of nonpenetrating procedures argue that with fewer potential complications, surgery may be considered earlier in the disease process, and that the target IOP may therefore not need to be as low.

Chai C, Loon SC. Meta-analysis of viscocanalostomy versus trabeculectomy in uncontrolled glaucoma. *J Glaucoma.* 2010;19(8):519–527.

Gilmour DF, Manners TD, Devonport H, Varga Z, Solebo AL, Miles J. Viscocanalostomy versus trabeculectomy for primary open angle glaucoma: 4-year prospective randomized clinical trial. *Eye.* 2009;23(9):1802–1807.

Lewis RA, Von Wolff K, Tetz M, et al. Canaloplasty: circumferential viscodilation and tensioning of Schlemm canal using a flexible microcatheter for the treatment of open-angle glaucoma in adults: 2-year interim clinical study results. *J Cataract Refract Surg.* 2009;35(5):814–824.

Sarodia U, Shaarawy T, Barton K. Nonpenetrating glaucoma surgery: a critical evaluation. *Curr Opin Ophthalmol.* 2007;18(2):152–158.

Schoenberg ED, Chaudhry AL, Chod R, Zurakowski D, Ayyala RS. Comparison of Surgical Outcomes between Phacocanaloplasty and Phacotrabeculectomy at 12 months' Follow-up: a Longitudinal Cohort Study. *J Glaucoma.* 2015;24(7):543–549.

Other Glaucoma Surgeries

The last decade saw the development of a number of devices that are used in surgical procedures to shunt aqueous from the anterior chamber directly into the Schlemm canal or the suprachoroidal space. These procedures, many of which require a gonioscopic view to perform, are considered minimally invasive and enhance the eye's natural aqueous outflow pathways. They are indicated in early to moderate open-angle glaucoma for patients who cannot tolerate or adhere to prescribed medication(s) and for patients for whom the risks of traditional surgeries may not be warranted. The procedures are frequently performed at the same time as cataract surgery but can be performed as standalone procedures.

Ab interno trabeculectomy is similar to goniotomy or ab externo trabeculotomy for pediatric eyes. Used in adult eyes, the procedure is performed with a disposable handpiece (Trabectome, NeoMedix) that fits through a clear corneal incision and delivers an electrosurgical pulse to remove trabecular meshwork, the anatomical site of greatest resistance to aqueous outflow. Electroablation of 180° of the trabecular meshwork (Video 8-7) allows aqueous to flow directly to the Schlemm canal and collector channels. Trabecular meshwork resistance also can be bypassed with a microshunt (iStent, Glaukos Corp). This device is a self-retaining titanium angled tube, which is placed into the Schlemm canal using a preloaded inserter (Video 8-8). Other microshunts and devices to remove trabecular meshwork are currently under development. These surgeries are indicated in open-angle glaucoma where trabecular meshwork is readily visible. Reflux bleeding and hyphemas are common postoperatively. There are no long-term prospective data on these procedures. Two-year data comparing a microshunt in combination with cataract surgery to cataract surgery alone showed a slightly higher rate of IOP maintenance below 21 mm Hg without medication in the combined surgery group.

 VIDEO 8-7 Trabectome: set up and procedure.
Courtesy of Sameh Mosaed, MD.

 VIDEO 8-8 iStent implantation.
Courtesy of Shakeel Shareef, MD.

Clinical trials evaluating aqueous shunting to the suprachoroidal space from an internal approach with various devices are currently under way. Suprachoroidal shunts used with an external approach and made of various materials were tried in the past but were unsuccessful because of problems with hypotony from cyclodialysis cleft formation or ocular hypertension, which developed as a result of scar formation at the posterior end of the seton.

Craven ER, Katz LJ, Wells JM, Giamporcaro JE; iStent Study Group. Cataract surgery with trabecular micro-bypass stent implantation in patients with mild-to-moderate open-angle glaucoma and cataracts: two-year follow-up. *J Cataract Refract Surg.* 2012;38(8):1339–1345.

Jea SY, Francis BA, Vakili G, Filippopoulos T, Rhee DJ. Ab interno trabeculectomy versus trabeculectomy for open-angle glaucoma. *Ophthalmology.* 2012;119(1):36–42.

Skaat A, Sagiv O, Kinori M, Simon GJ, Goldenfeld M, Melamed S. Gold Micro-Shunt Implants Versus Ahmed Glaucoma Valve: Long-term Outcomes of a Prospective Randomized Clinical Trial [epub ahead of print October 14, 2014]. *J Glaucoma.*

Incisional Surgeries Specific to Angle-Closure Glaucoma

Peripheral iridectomy

Surgical iridectomy may be required if a patent iridotomy cannot be achieved with laser in cases of pupillary block. Such situations include a cloudy cornea, a shallow or flat anterior chamber, and inadequate patient cooperation. Surgical iridectomy is performed through a clear corneal or scleral tunnel incision.

Chamber deepening and goniosynechialysis

When PAS develop in cases of acute angle closure, iridotomy alone may not lower the IOP adequately. Deepening the anterior chamber through a paracentesis may break PAS that are of relatively recent onset. *Goniosynechialysis,* a surgical procedure to break synechiae, is performed in the operating room alone or in combination with cataract surgery. Forceps, a blunt spatula, and/or a viscoelastic agent can be used for goniosynechialysis of PAS that are of less than 6–12 months' duration.

Campbell DG, Vela A. Modern goniosynechialysis for the treatment of synechial angle-closure glaucoma. *Ophthalmology.* 1984;91(9):1052–1060.

Shingleton BJ, Chang MA, Bellows AR, Thomas JV. Surgical goniosynechialysis for angle-closure glaucoma. *Ophthalmology.* 1990;97(5):551–556.

Special Considerations in the Surgical Management of Elderly Patients

When deciding whether to proceed with surgery in an elderly patient, the surgeon must take into account several issues specific to this population. The first issue is determining the appropriateness of surgery. The surgeon must consider the severity of the disease and the risk of functional vision loss in relation to the patient's life expectancy. Also, the surgeon must assess the patient's ability to adhere to medical therapy. A patient who is poorly adherent preoperatively (because of memory loss, poor vision, tremor, or arthritis) stands a high risk of being nonadherent in the postoperative phase and may well jeopardize the outcome as a result. In addition, the surgeon must consider whether the presence of a major systemic disease would affect the patient's ability to physically withstand the stress of surgery.

Once the decision has been made to proceed with surgery, the surgeon should determine which procedure is most likely to be successful and result in the fewest complications. The surgeon should consider the patient's ability to return to the clinic or office for multiple follow-up visits. If a patient is not mobile or has no easy transportation options, a nonpenetrating surgery or cyclodestructive procedure may be preferred, as these procedures require fewer postoperative visits than a trabeculectomy requires. If a trabeculectomy is decided upon, a limbus-based conjunctival flap is less likely to leak than a fornix-based flap and might be considered. The patient's use of anticoagulants and antiplatelet medications should also be evaluated, as the risk of serious complications from intraocular hemorrhage is increased with their use, and stopping these medications is associated with a risk of cerebrovascular events. Finally, the surgeon must factor in compromised healing in elderly persons and be circumspect about the use of antifibrotics in this group, whose tissues tend to be thinner and more fragile compared with younger patients.

Basic Texts

Glaucoma

Allingham RR, Damji KF, Freedman S, Maroi SE, Rhee DJ. *Shields' Textbook of Glaucoma.* 6th ed. Philadelphia: Lippincott Williams & Wilkins; 2010.

Anderson DR, Patella VM. *Automated Static Perimetry.* 2nd ed. St Louis: Mosby; 1998.

Epstein DL, Allingham RR, Schuman JS, eds. *Chandler and Grant's Glaucoma.* 4th ed. Baltimore: Lippincott Williams & Wilkins; 1997.

Levin LA, Nilsson SFE, Ver Hoeve J, Wu SM, Kaufman PL, Alm A. *Adler's Physiology of the Eye: Clinical Application.* 11th ed. New York: Saunders/Elsevier; 2011.

Ritch R, Shields MB, Krupin T, eds. *The Glaucomas.* 2nd ed. St Louis: Mosby; 1996.

Stamper RL, Lieberman MF, Drake MV, eds. *Becker-Shaffer's Diagnosis and Therapy of the Glaucomas.* 8th ed. St Louis: Mosby; 2009.

Tasman W, Jaeger EA, eds. *Duane's Ophthalmology on DVD-ROM.* Philadelphia: Lippincott Williams & Wilkins; 2012.

Weinreb RN, Mills RP, eds. *Glaucoma Surgery: Principles and Techniques.* 2nd ed. Ophthalmology Monographs 4. San Francisco: American Academy of Ophthalmology; 1998.

Zimmerman TJ, Kooner KS, Fechtner RD, Sharir M. *Textbook of Ocular Pharmacology.* 3rd ed. Philadelphia: Lippincott Williams & Wilkins; 1997.

Related Academy Materials

The American Academy of Ophthalmology is dedicated to providing a wealth of high-quality clinical education resources for ophthalmologists.

Print Publications and Electronic Products

For a complete listing of Academy products related to topics covered in this BCSC Section, visit our online store at http://store.aao.org/clinical-education/topic/glaucoma.html. Or call Customer Service at 866.561.8558 (toll free, US only) or +1 415.561.8540, Monday through Friday, between 8:00 AM and 5:00 PM (PST).

Online Resources

Visit the Ophthalmic News and Education (ONE®) Network at aao.org/onenetwork to find relevant videos, online courses, journal articles, practice guidelines, self-assessment quizzes, images and more. The ONE Network is a free Academy-member benefit.

Access free, trusted articles and content with the Academy's collaborative online encyclopedia, EyeWiki, at aao.org/eyewiki.

Requesting Continuing Medical Education Credit

The American Academy of Ophthalmology is accredited by the Accreditation Council for Continuing Medical Education (ACCME) to provide continuing medical education for physicians.

The American Academy of Ophthalmology designates this enduring material for a maximum of 10 *AMA PRA Category 1 Credits*™. Physicians should claim only the credit commensurate with the extent of their participation in the activity.

To claim *AMA PRA Category 1 Credits*™ upon completion of this activity, learners must demonstrate appropriate knowledge and participation in the activity by taking the posttest for Section 10 and achieving a score of 80% or higher.

This Section of the BCSC has been approved by the American Board of Ophthalmology as a Maintenance of Certification Part II self-assessment CME activity.

To take the posttest and request CME credit online:

1. Go to www.aao.org/cme-central and log in.
2. Click on "Claim CME Credit and View My CME Transcript" and then "Report AAO Credits."
3. Select the appropriate media type and then the Academy activity. You will be directed to the posttest.
4. Once you have passed the test with a score of 80% or higher, you will be directed to your transcript. *If you are not an Academy member, you will be able to print out a certificate of participation once you have passed the test.*

CME expiration date: June 1, 2020. *AMA PRA Category 1 Credits*™ may be claimed only once between June 1, 2016, and the expiration date.

For assistance, contact the Academy's Customer Service department at 866-561-8558 (US only) or +1 415-561-8540 between 8:00 AM and 5:00 PM (PST), Monday through Friday, or send an e-mail to customer_service@aao.org.

Study Questions

Please note that these questions are not part of your CME reporting process. They are provided here for your own educational use and identification of any professional practice gaps. The required CME posttest is available online (see "Requesting CME Credit"). Following the questions are a blank answer sheet and answers with discussions. Although a concerted effort has been made to avoid ambiguity and redundancy in these questions, the authors recognize that differences of opinion may occur regarding the "best" answer. The discussions are provided to demonstrate the rationale used to derive the answer. They may also be helpful in confirming that your approach to the problem was correct or, if necessary, in fixing the principle in your memory.

1. Prospective trials have found several risk factors for the development or progression of primary open-angle glaucoma (POAG). What factor is associated with a critical risk of progression in POAG?

    a. young age

    b. thicker cornea

    c. decreased perfusion pressure

    d. elevated intracranial pressure

2. What is the mode of inheritance of Axenfeld-Rieger syndrome?

    a. X-linked

    b. sporadic

    c. autosomal recessive

    d. autosomal dominant

3. Which parameter of the modified Goldmann equation cannot be directly measured clinically and must be calculated from the other parameters of this equation?

    a. outflow facility

    b. aqueous humor formation rate

    c. uveoscleral flow rate

    d. episcleral venous pressure

4. What is the rate of aqueous humor formation during sleep, compared with the rate during waking hours?

    a. the same as during waking hours

    b. decreased by approximately 50%

    c. increased by approximately 50%

    d. increased by 25%

5. What type of tonometer utilizes the Imbert-Fick principle for measurement of intraocular pressure (IOP)?

    a. pneumatonometer

    b. Schiøtz tonometer

    c. Perkins tonometer

    d. dynamic contour tonometer

6. When is a false-positive error recorded in perimetry?

    a. when the patient responds even though no visual stimulus was presented

    b. when the patient moves his or her eyes from the central fixation point

    c. when, on retesting, the patient does not respond to a stimulus that was previously seen

    d. when the patient falsely responds to a visual stimulus presented in the blind spot

7. What is the best way to examine the optic nerve head (also called optic disc) in routine clinical practice?

    a. with a slit-lamp biomicroscope and a high-magnification (eg, 60.00, 78.00, or 90.00 D) posterior pole lens

    b. with the indirect ophthalmoscope

    c. with the direct ophthalmoscope and low magnification

    d. with the direct ophthalmoscope and high magnification

8. What is the criterion that was used in the Ocular Hypertension Treatment Study (OHTS) for identification of a visual field defect on standard automated perimetry?

    a. presence of a Glaucoma Hemifield Test (GHT) with abnormally low sensitivity

    b. presence of a Pattern Standard Deviation (PSD) with $P < 5\%$ or presence of a GHT with a result outside normal limits

    c. presence of a cluster of 2 abnormal points on the pattern deviation plot

    d. diffuse loss of sensitivity with a mean deviation with $P < 5\%$

9. Mutations in which gene are associated with pseudoexfoliation syndrome?

    a. *CYP1B1*

    b. *FOXC1*

    c. *LOXL1*

    d. *PITX2*

10. What is the most common cause of glaucoma associated with primary or metastatic tumors of the ciliary body?

    a. angle closure by rotation of the ciliary body

    b. deposition of tumor cells and inflammatory cells in the trabecular meshwork

    c. direct invasion of the anterior chamber angle

    d. neovascularization of the angle

11. Which type of glaucoma is caused by leakage of lens protein through the capsule of a mature or hypermature cataract?

   a. phacomorphic glaucoma

   b. lens particle glaucoma

   c. ectopia lentis

   d. phacolytic glaucoma

12. In the assessment of a patient with acute bilateral angle closure and a normal axial length, what additional step is critical to reaching an accurate diagnosis?

   a. Perform an immediate bilateral paracentesis.

   b. Perform iris angiography.

   c. Take a medication history.

   d. Perform ultrasound biomicroscopy.

13. Peripheral iridotomy is the treatment of choice for what disorder?

   a. secondary angle closure following dense panretinal photocoagulation

   b. iridocorneal endothelial dystrophy

   c. phacoanaphylactic glaucoma

   d. phacomorphic glaucoma

14. What is the most important factor in determining when to perform a laser peripheral iridotomy in an eye with a narrow angle?

   a. gonioscopic findings

   b. amount of glaucomatous optic nerve cupping

   c. amount of glaucomatous visual field loss

   d. IOP level

15. What type of primary angle closure (PAC) occurs independent of pupillary block?

   a. acute PAC

   b. intermittent PAC

   c. plateau iris syndrome

   d. subacute PAC

16. What type of glaucoma is unlikely to resolve after cataract extraction?

   a. primary angle-closure glaucoma

   b. phacolytic glaucoma

   c. an eye with angle recession and phacodonesis after blunt trauma

   d. microspherophakia with glaucoma

17. What finding on examination of a patient with congenital glaucoma can continue to change and indicate progressive glaucoma even though the IOP appears to be controlled?

    a. axial length

    b. corneal thickness

    c. gonioscopic findings

    d. myopia

18. After successful surgery for congenital glaucoma, for how many years should a child be monitored?

    a. 5 years

    b. 10 years

    c. 20 years

    d. for life

19. What glaucoma medication is contraindicated in the treatment of glaucoma in a toddler?

    a. brimonidine

    b. dorzolamide

    c. latanoprost

    d. timolol

20. Which class of ocular hypotensive agents is associated with the development of apnea in infants and young children?

    a. α_2-selective adrenergic agonists

    b. nonselective β-antagonists

    c. carbonic anhydrase inhibitors

    d. cholinergic agonists

21. Compared with nonselective adrenergic antagonists, which topical β_1-selective adrenergic antagonist is less likely to induce bronchospasm in patients with mild asthma?

    a. timolol

    b. carteolol

    c. betaxolol

    d. levobunolol

22. In a patient undergoing trabeculectomy for a preoperative IOP of 50 mm Hg, which crystalline lens status and postoperative IOP level pose the greatest risk for development of a suprachoroidal hemorrhage?

    a. phakic eye with a postoperative IOP in the mid teens

    b. phakic eye with a postoperative IOP in the single digits

    c. aphakic eye with a postoperative IOP in the mid teens

    d. aphakic eye with a postoperative IOP in the single digits

23. Five years after laser trabeculoplasty, what percentage of treated patients are expected to maintain a lower IOP?

   a. 20%

   b. 30%

   c. 40%

   d. 50%

24. Who is the best candidate for a trabeculectomy with mitomycin C?

   a. aphakic contact lens wearer

   b. patient with neovascular glaucoma

   c. patient with previous failed trabeculectomy without antifibrotics

   d. patient with active uveitis

25. What patient profile has the most success with laser trabeculoplasty?

   a. aphakic patient who is intolerant of multiple medications and whose current IOP is above the target pressure

   b. patient with a 10° central island of vision who is on maximally tolerated core medical therapy

   c. patient with POAG who is intolerant of multiple medications and whose current IOP is above the target pressure

   d. patient with uveitic glaucoma

Answer Sheet for Section 10 Study Questions

Question	Answer	Question	Answer
1	a b c d	14	a b c d
2	a b c d	15	a b c d
3	a b c d	16	a b c d
4	a b c d	17	a b c d
5	a b c d	18	a b c d
6	a b c d	19	a b c d
7	a b c d	20	a b c d
8	a b c d	21	a b c d
9	a b c d	22	a b c d
10	a b c d	23	a b c d
11	a b c d	24	a b c d
12	a b c d	25	a b c d
13	a b c d		

Answers

1. **c.** In prospective trials, decreased perfusion pressure, thinner cornea, and increasing age have been shown to be important risk factors for progression of glaucoma. Intracranial pressure may have an effect on the translaminar pressure gradient but has not been studied in clinical trials. Furthermore, lower intracranial pressure has been implicated as a factor in low-tension glaucoma but has not been explored in a longitudinal trial.

2. **d.** Axenfeld-Rieger syndrome is an autosomal dominant disorder and presents with a variety of phenotypes.

3. **c.** Outflow facility is measured with tonography; aqueous humor formation rate, with fluorophotometry; and episcleral venous pressure, with venomanometry. All of these procedures are noninvasive. In contrast, direct measurement of uveoscleral flow rate is an invasive process that involves perfusion of a tracer into the anterior segment of the eye, followed by estimation of the tissue distribution of the tracer. Thus, in humans, uveoscleral outflow rate must be calculated by using the Goldmann equation and the parameters intraocular pressure (IOP), aqueous humor flow rate, outflow facility, and episcleral venous pressure.

4. **b.** During waking hours, the rate of aqueous humor formation is normally about 2–3 μL/min. During sleep, the rate decreases by approximately 50%. There are no known cases of glaucoma that are caused by overproduction of aqueous humor.

5. **c.** Like the Goldmann tonometer, the Perkins tonometer is an applanation tonometer and, as such, is based on the Imbert-Fick principle. The Imbert-Fick principle relates the pressure inside a dry, thin-walled sphere to the force required to flatten a specific area. The Goldmann applanation tonometer and the Perkins tonometer use the same measurement tip, which balances surface tension of the tear film with the rigidity of the cornea to approximate a dry, infinitely flexible, thin-walled sphere for eyes with corneal thickness of 520 μm.

6. **a.** A false-positive occurs when the patient presses the button and shows a response without presentation of any visual stimulus.

7. **a.** A slit-lamp biomicroscope and a high-magnification posterior pole lens allow stereoscopic and detailed routine examination of the optic nerve head. The direct ophthalmoscope also may be used for clinical examination of the optic nerve head. However, this instrument may not provide sufficient stereoscopic detail to detect subtle changes in optic nerve head topography. Indirect ophthalmoscopy provides a low-magnification view that is insufficient for detailed examination.

8. **b.** In the Ocular Hypertension Treatment Study (OHTS), a visual field defect was defined as the presence of a Pattern Standard Deviation (PSD) with $P < 5\%$ or the presence of a Glaucoma Hemifield Test (GHT) with a result outside normal limits; the abnormality had to be present in 3 consecutive visual field tests.

9. **c.** *CYP1B1* is associated with primary congenital glaucoma; *FOXC1,* with iridogoniodysgenesis; and *PITX2,* with Rieger syndrome. Pseudoexfoliation syndrome is associated with *LOXL1* mutations at 15q24.

10. **c.** While choices a, b, and d may all cause glaucoma associated with primary or metastatic tumors of the ciliary body, direct invasion of the anterior chamber angle is the most common cause in these cases.

11. **d.** In a mature or hypermature cataract, soluble lens protein molecules are released through microscopic openings in the lens capsule into the anterior chamber. Secondary open-angle glaucoma (OAG) may develop as lens proteins, phagocytizing macrophages, and other inflammatory debris obstruct the trabecular meshwork. Medications should be used to treat the IOP elevation; however, definitive therapy requires cataract extraction.

    In phacomorphic glaucoma, a large, intumescent lens induces angle-closure glaucoma (ACG). Lens particle glaucoma occurs when lens cortex particles obstruct the trabecular meshwork following disruption of the lens capsule with cataract extraction or ocular trauma. Ectopia lentis refers to displacement of the lens from its normal anatomical position.

12. **c.** Bilateral angle closure is not common and is especially uncommon in eyes with a normal axial length. The presentation of bilateral angle closure should strongly suggest uveal effusions due to use of a systemic medication, most commonly topiramate.

13. **d.** Laser iridotomy is useful for treating angle closure when there is an element of pupillary block (eg, as in phacomorphic glaucoma). Iridotomy is of no benefit when angle closure is caused by other mechanisms and may exacerbate the condition if outflow is further diminished by the inflammation that usually occurs as a result of the procedure.

14. **a.** In chronic primary angle closure (PAC) with relative pupillary block, gonioscopic findings are the key to diagnosis and management. IOP may be normal or elevated. In an eye with a narrow angle, the presence of elevated pressure alone is not an indication for laser iridotomy. In this case, coexisting OAG may be causing the IOP elevation, not the narrow angle. The extent of visual field loss or optic nerve damage does not indicate whether an iridotomy is needed. In patients with appositional angle closure or areas of peripheral anterior synechiae with relative pupillary block, the risk of chronic angle closure developing is high; thus, these patients should have a laser iridotomy.

15. **c.** Elevation of IOP occurs with plateau iris syndrome independent of pupillary block and may occur despite a patent iridotomy.

16. **c.** Cataract extraction would not be expected to improve control of IOP in an eye with blunt trauma and direct trabecular damage. Angle recession may be present and would be evidence of trabecular damage. Phacodonesis is evidence of zonular disruption. In this patient, the lens is not contributing to the IOP elevation. In chronic primary ACG, relative pupillary block is induced by the tension of the iris sphincter muscle against the lens, which is positioned slightly anteriorly, in an eye with a relatively short axial length. Cataract surgery may improve glaucoma control or may completely eliminate glaucoma in these eyes. In phacolytic glaucoma, proteinaceous lens material that is released through microscopic openings in the lens capsule and engulfed by macrophages clogs the trabecular meshwork and causes secondary elevation of IOP. Cataract surgery may successfully treat this form of glaucoma. In microspherophakia, the abnormal, spherical shape of the lens induces pupillary block, which a laser peripheral iridotomy or lens removal would be expected to relieve.

17. **a.** In children younger than 3 years, the sclera is elastic and will stretch if IOP is not well controlled. This can result in increased axial length despite a good pressure during ex-

amination under anesthesia. Corneal thickness decreases as corneal edema resolves and, once stable, is often less than the average central corneal thickness. The angle can further develop as a child ages, but this does not indicate poor pressure control. Myopia in congenital glaucoma is not necessarily an axial myopia.

18. **d.** Patients with congenital glaucoma require lifelong monitoring, as relapses may occur even decades after initial surgery. These patients may also have postoperative complications, amblyopia, strabismus, corneal decompensation, cataracts, and other problems that will need to be managed over a lifetime.

19. **a.** Brimonidine has been shown to cause systemic hypotension and apnea in children younger than 2 years. This drug is relatively contraindicated in older children.

20. **a.** α_2-Selective adrenergic agonists have been reported to cause severe, life-threatening apnea, central nervous system depression, and bradycardia in infants and children. These agents can cross the blood–brain barrier, particularly in infants. They are contraindicated for use in young children and should be avoided in nursing mothers.

21. **c.** Timolol, carteolol, and levobunolol are nonselective β-adrenergic antagonists (β-blockers). β_2 receptors are present in bronchial smooth muscle cells, where their inhibition may result in bronchospasm. The only topical ocular hypotensive β-blocker that is relatively β_1 selective is betaxolol; it is thus less likely to result in pulmonary adverse effects. The nonselective agents are more effective in lowering IOP than is betaxolol.

22. **d.** Suprachoroidal hemorrhage can be one of the most devastating complications of trabeculectomy. Bleeding originates from the short or long posterior ciliary arteries as they enter the suprachoroidal space from the intrascleral canal. Delayed suprachoroidal hemorrhage is usually preceded by hypotony and the development of serous ciliochoroidal effusions, which stretch and rupture one of the vessels where the vessel bridges the suprachoroidal space.

Conditions associated with an increased risk of suprachoroidal hemorrhage include high myopia, aphakia or pseudophakia, hypotony, prior vitrectomy, advanced age, systemic hypertension, anticoagulant therapy, and history of suprachoroidal hemorrhage in the fellow eye. The Fluorouracil Filtering Surgery Study found that the risk of suprachoroidal hemorrhage was strongly associated with the level of preoperative IOP and the magnitude of IOP reduction. Reducing the IOP as much as possible before filtering surgery and decreasing the magnitude of the immediate IOP reduction through the use of releasable sutures or laser suture lysis can help reduce the risk of this complication.

23. **d.** Studies show that 3–5 years following laser trabeculoplasty, 50% of treated patients have a lower IOP.

24. **c.** All of these patients are good candidates for a tube shunt, as all patients listed have indications for a tube shunt. However, the patient who previously had a failed trabeculectomy without antifibrotics is the one most likely to have a successful trabeculectomy with mitomycin C. The Fluorouracil Filtering Surgery Study found that use of 5-fluorouracil increases the likelihood of success of a trabeculectomy, and subsequent studies have found that mitomycin C increases success rates more than 5-fluorouracil does.

An aphakic patient is likely to have scleral scarring from surgery to remove the cataract, and contact lens wear is a risk factor for bleb-related infections. Neovascular glaucoma and uveitic glaucoma are associated with inflammation, which lowers the success rate of trabeculectomy with or without antifibrotic use.

25. **c.** Laser trabeculoplasty (LTP) can be used as primary or adjunct therapy in patients with open angles. If the pressure needs to be lowered but the patient cannot tolerate multiple medications, LTP is a good option. LTP is less effective in aphakic and pseudophakic patients than in phakic patients. A patient with a small central island of vision who is on maximally tolerated medical therapy is at risk of vision loss if there is a significant IOP spike. LTP is contraindicated in uveitic glaucoma, because the angle is altered in eyes with a history of inflammation and studies have shown low success rates in these patients.

Index

(*f* = figure; *t* = table)